Curbside
Consultation
in Pediatric Dermatology

Curbside Consultation in Pediatrics
SERIES

SERIES EDITOR, LISA B. ZAOUTIS

Curbside Consultation
in Pediatric Dermatology

Editor

James R. Treat, MD

Assistant Professor of Pediatrics and Dermatology
Perelman School of Medicine
University of Pennsylvania
Children's Hospital of Philadelphia
Philadelphia, Pennsylvania

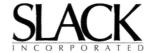

SLACK
INCORPORATED

www.Healio.com/books

ISBN: 978-1-61711-003-0

Published by: SLACK Incorporated
                   6900 Grove Road
                   Thorofare, NJ 08086 USA
                   Telephone: 856-848-1000
                   Fax: 856-848-6091
                   www.Healio.com/books

Contact SLACK Incorporated for more information about other books in this field or about the availability of our books from distributors outside the United States.

Library of Congress Cataloging-in-Publication Data

Curbside consultation in pediatric dermatology : 49 clinical questions / editor, James Treat.
     p. ; cm. -- (Curbside consultation in pediatrics series)
  Pediatric dermatology
  Includes bibliographical references.
  ISBN 978-1-61711-003-0 (pbk. : alk. paper)
  I. Treat, James (James R.) II. Title: Pediatric dermatology. III. Series: Curbside consultation in pediatrics series.
  [DNLM: 1. Skin diseases--therapy. 2. Child. 3. Infant. 4. Skin diseases diagnosis. WS 260]
  LC classification not assigned
  618.92'5 dc23
                                   2012006220

Printed in the United States of America.

Last digit is print number: 10   9   8   7   6   5   4   3   2   1

Dedication

I dedicate this book to my wonderful wife and our 2 amazing children who provide the inspiration, comic relief, and joy that make our lives.

Contents

Acknowledgments

I thank Dr. Paul J. Honig, Dr. Albert C. Yan, and Dr. D. William James whose incredible patient care and wisdom I will always try to emulate.

About the Editor

James R. Treat, MD is an assistant professor of Pediatrics and Dermatology at the Perelman School of Medicine at the University of Pennsylvania in Philadelphia, with his major clinical appointment at the Children's Hospital of Philadelphia.

Contributing Authors

Faizan Alawi, DDS (Question 15)
Associate Professor
Department of Pathology
School of Dental Medicine
Department of Dermatology
School of Medicine
University of Pennsylvania
Philadelphia, Pennsylvania

Lisa Arkin, MD (Questions 9, 25, 34)
Resident
Department of Dermatology
Northwestern University
Feinberg School of Medicine
Chicago, Illinois

Terri Brown-Whitehorn, MD (Question 29)
Assistant Professor of Clinical Pediatrics
Perelman School of Medicine
University of Pennsylvania
Philadelphia, Pennsylvania

John C. Browning, MD, FAAD, FAAP
   (Questions 16, 22, 35)
Chief
Pediatric Dermatology
Assistant Professor of Pediatrics and
   Dermatology
University of Texas Health Science Center
San Antonio, Texas

Leslie Castelo-Soccio, MD, PhD (Questions 11,
   13, 17, 40, 41)
Assistant Professor of Pediatrics and
   Dermatology
Perelman School of Medicine
University of Pennsylvania
The Children's Hospital of Philadelphia
Philadelphia, Pennsylvania

Glen H. Crawford, MD (Question 24)
Chief of Dermatology
Pennsylvania Hospital
Clinical Associate Professor
Department of Dermatology
Perelman School of Medicine
University of Pennsylvania
Philadelphia, Pennsylvania

Bhavik S. Desai, DMD, PhD (Question 15)
Resident
Oral Medicine
Hospital of University of Pennsylvania
Philadelphia, Pennsylvania

Magdalene Dohil, MD (Questions 4, 8, 42)
Associate Professor of Clinical Pediatrics
   and Medicine (Dermatology)
University of California, San Diego
Rady Children's Hospital
San Diego, California

Lawrence F. Eichenfield, MD (Questions 4,
   8, 42)
Professor of Clinical Pediatrics and
   Medicine (Dermatology)
Chief
Pediatric and Adolescent Dermatology
University of California
San Diego School of Medicine
Rady Children's Hospital
San Diego, California

Dirk M. Elston, MD (Questions 19, 33, 47)
Director
Ackerman Academy of Dermatopathology
Clinical Professor of Dermatology
New York College of Osteopathic Medicine
New York, New York

Brian T. Fisher, DO, MSCE, MPH
  (Question 37)
Assistant Professor of Pediatrics
Perelman School of Medicine
University of Pennsylvania
Philadelphia, Pennsylvania

Ilona J. Frieden, MD (Questions 1, 2)
Professor of Dermatology and Pediatrics
Departments of Dermatology
University of California
San Francisco, California

Sheila F. Friedlander, MD (Questions 31, 32)
Professor of Clinical Pediatrics and
  Medicine
University of California San Diego
  School of Medicine
Rady Children's Hospital
San Diego, California

Maj. Sarah M. Frioux, MD (Questions 38, 39)
Major, US Army Medical Corps
Child Abuse Pediatrician
Tripler Army Medical Center
Honolulu, Hawaii
Assistant Professor of Pediatrics
Uniformed Services University of the
  Health Sciences
F. Edward Hebert School of Medicine
Honolulu, Hawaii

Maria C. Garzon, MD (Question 3)
Professor of Clinical Dermatology and
  Clinical Pediatrics
Columbia University
New York, New York

Warren R. Heymann, MD (Questions 44, 46, 49)
Head
Division of Dermatology
Professor of Medicine and Pediatrics
Cooper Medical School of Rowan University
Camden, New Jersey

Sharon E. Jacob, MD (Question 24)
Associate Clinical Professor
Medicine and Pediatrics (Dermatology-WOS)
University of California
San Diego, California

Christine T. Lauren, MD (Question 5)
Assistant Professor of Clinical
Dermatology and Clinical Pediatrics
Columbia University Medical Center
New York, New York

Moise L. Levy, MD (Questions 6, 14)
Clinical Professor, Dermatology and
  Pediatrics
Baylor College of Medicine
Clinical Professor of Dermatology
University of Texas Southwestern
  Medical School
Dell Children's Medical Center
Austin, Texas

Erin F. Mathes, MD (Questions 1, 2)
Assistant Clinical Professor of
  Dermatology and Pediatrics
University of California
San Francisco, California

Patrick McMahon, MD (Questions 7, 12, 30)
Pediatric Dermatology Fellow
The Children's Hospital of Philadelphia
Philadelphia, Pennsylvania

Christopher J. Miller, MD (Question 48)
Director of Dermatologic Surgery
Assistant Professor of Dermatology
University of Pennsylvania
Perelman Center for Advanced Medicine
Philadelphia, Pennsylvania

Kimberly D. Morel, MD, FAAD, FAAP
  (Question 23)
Associate Professor of Clinical
Dermatology and Clinical Pediatrics
Columbia University/Morgan Stanley
  Children's Hospital of New York
  Presbyterian
New York, New York

Adam Nabatian, MD (Question 44)
Resident
Department of Dermatology
Albert Einstein College of Medicine
New York, New York

Marissa J. Perman, MD (Questions 27, 43, 45)
Pediatric Dermatology Fellow
Children's Hospital of Philadelphia
Philadelphia, Pennsylvania

*Andres Pinto, DMD, MPH, FDS RCSEd
   (Question 15)*
Associate Professor of Oral Medicine
Associate Professor of Community Health
Director of Oral Medicine Services
Division Chief
Community Oral Health
University of Pennsylvania
Robert Schattner Center School of Dental
   Medicine
Philadelphia, Pennsylvania

Anna S. Salinas, MD (Questions 6, 14)
Le Bonheur Children's Hospital
Clinical Professor of Dermatology and
   Pediatrics
Baylor College of Medicine
Clinical Professor of Dermatology
University of Texas Southwestern
   Medical School
Physician-in-Chief
Dell Children's Medical Center
Austin, Texas

Kara N. Shah, MD, PhD (Question 10)
Director
Division of Pediatric Dermatology
Cincinnati Children's Hospital
Associate Professor of Pediatrics and
   Dermatology
University of Cincinnati College of
   Medicine
Cincinnati, Ohio

Randy Tang, MD (Questions 46, 49)
University of Medicine and Dentistry,
   New Jersey-Robert Wood Johnson
   Medical School
Department of Dermatology
Cooper University Hospital
Camden, New Jersey

Joanne Wood, MD, MSHP (Questions 38, 39)
Child Abuse Pediatrics Fellowship
   Program Director
Children's Hospital of Philadelphia
Philadelphia, Pennsylvania

*Albert C. Yan, MD, FAAP, FAAD
   (Questions 18, 36)*
Chief
Pediatric Dermatology
Associate Professor of Pediatrics and
   Dermatology
Perelman School of Medicine
University of Pennsylvania
Children's Hospital of Philadelphia
Philadelphia, Pennsylvania

Andrea L. Zaenglein, MD (Questions 20, 21, 28)
Associate Professor of Dermatology and
   Pediatrics
Penn State Milton S. Hershey Medical
   Center
Hershey, Pennsylvania

Preface

This book is inspired by the fantastic patient-care questions I consistently receive from both pediatric practitioners and dermatologists. This book is a compilation of the most commonly asked questions that will hopefully make the biggest positive impact on the care of skin problems in pediatric patients. Skin complaints are one of the most common medical issues in the pediatric patient and the questions answered in this book specifically help with everyday management of both common and life-threatening conditions, with a concentration on diagnostic differentiation and therapeutic management. We have compiled practical tips that help with everyday decisions so that the practitioner can see the forest through the trees when diagnosing and treating skin issues. There are some off-label recommendations in this book because many pediatric skin diseases do not have FDA-approved options but still need to have their diseases treated. These recommendations must be evaluated and adapted in the context of a specific patient scenario to see if they are reasonable for any individual decisions. This book aims to provide a straightforward and thoughtful approach to the diagnosis and management of common pediatric skin diseases. The chapters are organized based on the way patients actually present to practitioners by asking and then answering the most common questions we get as pediatric dermatologists.

Foreword

We were sitting together on a plane after lecturing at a CME course, on our way back to Philadelphia. Jim Treat asked, "What questions do referring physicians (especially pediatricians) frequently ask you about?" "Are you planning another talk?" I replied. "No," he said, "I want to put something together about pediatric dermatology that would be helpful for pediatricians, family physicians, and dermatologists who don't see a lot of kids." He stated his aim was to give physicians practical clinical insight on how to approach skin conditions they see in their pediatric patients. I can only surmise that is when the concept of *Curbside Consultation in Pediatric Dermatology: 49 Clinical Questions* took place. For sure Jim would be perfect for this project because of his uncanny teaching skills.

What can I tell you about Dr. Treat (who I have known since he started his dermatology residency at Penn)? He is young (early in his career in pediatric dermatology), smart (top of his medical school class), and boy can he teach (the number of teaching award plaques on the wall of his office is amazing). Let me put it this way, at times attendings at our clinic are annoyed that the medical students and residents prefer to work with Jim. He is just a natural at conveying information to others. He has a knack of knowing what his audience desires. The fact that he is so good with kids and their parents also amazes me. Why? One has to consider the fact that he did an internal medicine internship and then practiced adult dermatology for several years before he came to us as a pediatric dermatology fellow at the Children's Hospital of Philadelphia. Of course we got him up to speed (gave him the pediatric perspective) with weekly well-baby clinics once per week for 6 months. Having 2 wonderful children of his own didn't hurt either.

Now you know how I feel about Dr. Treat; but what about the fruits of his efforts, this book? I have always felt a physician needs to know the *essential facts* about a condition (eg, only 1% of sebaceous nevi develop a malignancy; the risks of general anesthesia for young infants differ at a general hospital compared to a children's hospital), the clues on physical examination that help to diagnose a particular skin change (eg, the yellow, flat, raised, or verrucous surface of a sebaceous nevus, and a surface devoid of hair), and, of course, the treatment options as well as nuances of management (eg, pros and cons of surgical removal, age of patient when a sebaceous nevus should or should not be removed, cosmetic and psychological ramifications from both a child's or parent's perspective). Lastly, physicians like the information to be concise and to the point, with as little embellishments as possible. In the main, this book accomplishes these stated characteristics.

My most favorite section is the one on dermatitis (Section IV), the condition seen most frequently by practitioners. The other excellent sections include III (Rashes), V (Infections), and VIII (Other). I also liked Questions 1, 2, and 3 (hemangiomas); 5 (midline lesions); 9 (sunscreens); 40 (vitiligo); and 43 (acne). Finally, another positive will be the ease with which practitioners can scan the contents page to find the questions they will want help with.

Paul J. Honig, MD
Emeritus Professor of Pediatrics and Dermatology
University of Pennsylvania School of Medicine
Senior Physician
The Children's Hospital of Philadelphia
Philadelphia, Pennsylvania

Introduction

This book targets pediatric practitioners and dermatologists who take care of children on a daily basis. The chapters are written by many of the experts in the field who have incredible experience and have helped to develop the standards of care for various dermatologic conditions. This book covers many of the most commonly encountered skin issues of children and concentrates on the management questions we as practitioners commonly encounter. The book is written in a conversational style so that the patient-care tips are highlighted and very accessible. There are tables, diagrams, hierarchical therapeutic breakdowns, and pictures that help to organize the information in the most usable way possible. Although the title of each chapter is a very specific question, the answers cover a range of topics that must be addressed when contemplating the title question. The simple diagnostic and therapeutic tips in the chapters will help to augment the care of pediatric skin disease by even the most seasoned practitioner.

SECTION I

BIRTHMARKS/VASCULAR AND OTHER SKIN LESIONS

WHAT IS THE NATURAL PROGRESSION OF INFANTILE HEMANGIOMAS?

Erin F. Mathes, MD and Ilona J. Frieden, MD

Infantile hemangiomas (IHs) are the most common tumor of infancy, occurring in approximately 4% of infants. IHs are more common in females, preterm infants, multiple gestation pregnancies, and infants of mothers older than 30 years. Caucasian race is also a risk factor. IHs are made of small, immature blood vessels. In superficial hemangiomas, the blood vessels involve the upper dermis and lead to a bright strawberry red color. Deep hemangiomas involve the deep dermis and subcutis and are skin color to blue. Mixed hemangiomas—those that involve both superficial and deeper skin structures—have both features. IH have a unique natural history: they are flat or inapparent at birth, with a period of rapid growth during early infancy followed by gradual involution. Because of IHs' characteristic growth pattern, the clinical history is one of the most important keys to diagnosing an IH. In addition, because IHs undergo early, rapid growth, it is important to refer patients with potentially complicated IH sooner rather than later.

When evaluating a child with a possible IH, ask if it was visible the day the child was born; if it has changed since birth; if it is still growing, stable, or shrinking in size; and if it is growing proportionately or disproportionately with child's somatic growth. If there was an actual lump or thickening present the day the child was born, question the diagnosis of IH since this could represent another type of soft tissue growth such as a so-called rapidly involuting congenital hemangioma or other soft tissue neoplasm such as a kaposiform hemangioendothelioma or fibrosarcoma.

The very first sign of an IH (a premonitory or precursor mark) sometimes presents at or shortly after birth as a discoloration of the skin—a persistent red spot, an area of pallor, telangiectasias, or a bruise that initially may be attributed to perinatal trauma. The more easily recognizable superficial proliferative phase of IH is often noticed within the first few weeks of life. The initial shape of the hemangioma (either the precursor lesion or the early proliferative phase) typically has the shape and configuration of the fully grown hemangioma (Figure 1-1). IHs "mark out their territory" early in life, and once that territory is delineated, growth is volumetric rather than radial.

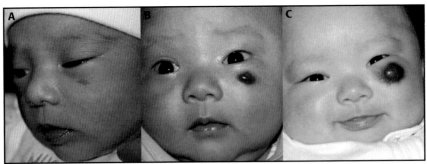

Figure 1-1. (A) Localized IH premonitory mark on the cheek of a 12-day-old infant. (B) Early growth at 49 days old. (C) The same IH at 2.3 months old—note the volumetric growth in essentially the same territory as the premonitory mark in (A).

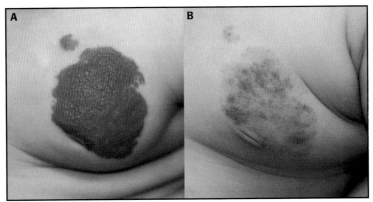

Figure 1-2. (A) Superficial IH on the breast of a 5-month-old infant. (B) Early involution—lightening and thinning—of the same IH.

For most IHs, the period of most rapid growth is between 4 and 6 weeks. In this time period, some IHs grow alarmingly quickly—doubling in size over a period of 1 to 2 weeks. Superficial hemangiomas typically become bright strawberry red and thicken, and sometimes become tense and shiny. Deep hemangiomas may be noted at a somewhat later age, on average 1 month later than superficial IHs, and occasionally not until a few months of life. Rapidly growing, deep hemangiomas often feel warm and slightly firm. As they proliferate, deep IHs increase in volume, and may develop more superficial telangiectasias, but they do not develop a superficial component if there was none to begin with. Once they have fully proliferated, deep IHs soften and become more doughy on palpation.

Contrary to what we used to believe about the growth of IH, we now know that 80% of growth is completed by 3 months of age and 80% of hemangiomas have actually stopped growing by 5 months of age. Large, segmental, deep, and parotid gland hemangiomas may have a prolonged growth phase (growing on average 1 month longer than superficial IHs).

Although the growth phase is usually weeks to months in duration, involution tends to be much slower, varying in length from months to years. Signs of involution include a change to a dull red, then gray or milky white color, flattening, softening, and ultimately a decrease in volume. Evidence of involution is usually apparent by 1 year of age (Figure 1-2). Smaller hemangiomas typically involute sooner than very large ones, but there are exceptions. Most IHs have involuted completely by the age of 7 to 10 years.

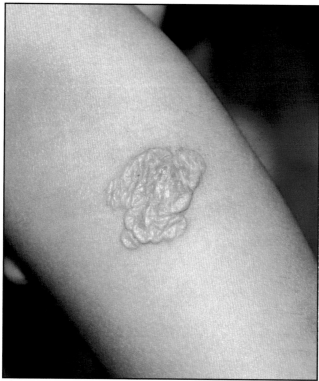

Figure 1-3. Residual fibrofatty tissue and anetoderma after involution of a superficial IH on the arm of a 4-year-old boy.

Unfortunately, involution does not equal resolution: a significant minority of children have residual skin changes such as telangiectasias, textural changes, fibrofatty residuum, or scars (Figure 1-3). The risk that an IH will leave behind cosmetically significant abnormalities is determined in part by location (eg, nasal tip, vermillion border, midcheek, ear, glabella, and periocular skin). In addition, hemangiomas in which the "strawberry" component is very thick, has a very exophytic superficial component with a steep slope, or a pedunculated or sessile shape are more likely to leave textural changes and fibrofatty tissue after involution. Ulcerated IHs virtually always cause scarring in the affected area of ulceration. Even small IHs in the locations, or with the characteristics mentioned above, should be referred early for consideration of treatment (see Question 2).

Growth characteristics of IHs help determine the timing and need for repeat evaluations in young infants: those with higher risk features, such as facial location, segmental distribution, and large size, with the potential to compromise function or cause significant disfigurement (see Question 2) should be evaluated early and followed at frequent intervals (every few weeks). Parents should be advised to call if the IH changes rapidly so that treatment can be initiated if necessary.

Suggested Readings

Brandling-Bennett HA, Metry DW, Baselga E, et al. Infantile hemangiomas with unusually prolonged growth phase: a case series. *Arch Dermatol.* 2008;144(12):1632-1637.

Bruckner AL, Frieden IJ. Hemangiomas of infancy. *J Am Acad Dermatol.* 2003;48(4):477-493.

Chang LC, Haggstrom AN, Drolet BA, et al. Growth characteristics of infantile hemangiomas: implications for management. *Pediatrics.* 2008;122(2):360-367.

ARE THERE TYPES OR LOCATIONS OF HEMANGIOMAS THAT REQUIRE SPECIAL ATTENTION?

Erin F. Mathes, MD and Ilona J. Frieden, MD

Although the majority of infantile hemangiomas (IHs) resolve without problems, a significant minority cause medical morbidities or leave permanent skin changes that can be quite disfiguring. *Anatomic location* and *subtype* of IHs best predict the risk of complication and need for early referral and treatment (Table 2-1). IHs can be classified as superficial (bright, strawberry red color), deep (skin color to blue), or mixed. In addition, IHs can be classified as localized (as if arising from one central focus), segmental (corresponding to a portion of a developmental segment or broad anatomic territory; Figure 2-1), or multifocal (usually multiple localized IHs).

Risk Zones

ANATOMIC LOCATION

Anatomic location is one of the most important factors affecting risk. Hemangiomas involving the central face (including the nose and perioral skin), periocular area, neck, mandibular region, and perineum should alert clinicians to possible increased risk of complications. In addition, patients with multiple or segmental IHs have a higher risk of extracutaneous disease. If possible, patients with the high-risk types of IHs described next should be referred to appropriate specialists early and followed closely, particularly during the proliferative phase. Early treatment can prevent complications and improve the child's ultimate functional and cosmetic outcome.

Face

IHs of the face (especially large and deep IHs) can cause permanent disfigurement by stretching the skin and disrupting important cosmetic units. The nasal tip and ear can be particularly problematic because the hemangioma distorts the early growth of these

7

Table 2-1
Features of High-Risk Infantile Hemangiomas and Recommended Evaluation

Anatomic Location/ Morphology	Associated Risk	Recommended Evaluation*
Facial, large segmental	PHACE syndrome (posterior fossa malformations, hemangiomas, arterial anomalies, cardiac defects, eye abnormalities, sternal clefting)	Echocardiogram Ophthalmology evaluation MRI/MRA of the brain and neck
Nasal tip, ear, large facial (especially with prominent dermal component)	Permanent scarring, disfigurement	
Periorbital and retrobulbar	Ocular axis occlusion, astigmatism, amblyopia, tear-duct occlusion	Ophthalmology evaluation
Segmental "beard area," central neck	Airway hemangioma	Otolaryngology referral
Perioral	Ulceration, disfigurement, feeding difficulties	
Segmental overlying lumbosacral spine	Tethered spinal cord, genitourinary anomalies	MRI of lumbosacral spine, consider renal ultrasound
Perineal, axilla, neck, perioral	Ulceration	
Multiple hemangiomas (>5)	Visceral involvement (especially liver, gastrointestinal tract), hypothyroidism	Liver ultrasound; if liver hemangiomas are present obtain TSH, T4, reverse T3

MRA indicates magnetic resonance angiography; MRI, magnetic resonance imaging; TSH, thyroid-stimulating hormone

*In addition to evaluation by Pediatric Dermatology or other specialists.

delicate structures and can cause permanent changes in the cartilage. IHs of the nose and ear can also ulcerate, sometimes deeply, leading to loss of cartilage.

Periocular Hemangiomas

Hemangiomas in the periocular area can cause visual problems via direct pressure on the eye or mass effect (Figure 2-2). This can lead to anisometropia (unequal refractive power in the two eyes) and amblyopia (partial or complete loss of vision in one eye), which, if untreated in an infant, can lead to permanent visual loss. Direct pressure on the cornea can cause astigmatism or myopia. Mass effect of the tumor itself can cause ptosis, proptosis, visual axis occlusion, strabismus, or tear duct occlusion. Any patient with a hemangioma in the periocular area should have a prompt formal ophthalmologic evaluation with repeat visits during the proliferative phase (typically the first 3 to 4 months of life).

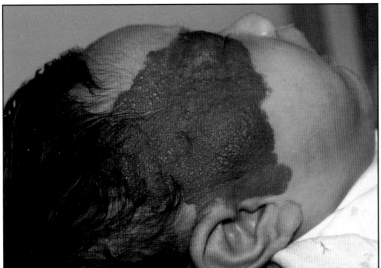

Figure 2-1. A superficial, segmental IH on the face of a 5-week-old girl.

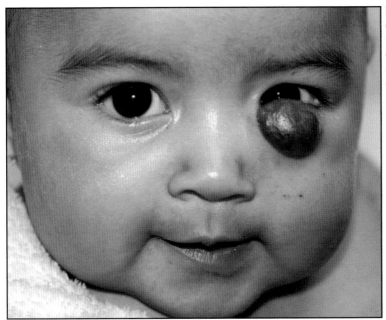

Figure 2-2. A 4-month-old girl with a localized, periocular IH that resulted in astigmatism and amblyopia. She was treated with prednisone followed by propranolol.

Perioral Hemangiomas

Perioral hemangiomas require special attention for two reasons: their potential for permanently distorting anatomic landmarks and their increased risk of ulceration. The lips have many curves, contours, and boundaries that can be easily distorted by the hemangioma mass, leaving permanent skin changes. Hemangiomas in this area are also more likely to ulcerate because of the moisture and repeated slight trauma associated with feeding and drooling. If a patient develops a lip ulceration, it can be painful enough to disrupt feeding and will always result in a scar. We recommend keeping all perioral IHs lubricated with petrolatum or a similar emollient to prevent trauma to the fragile skin.

Figure 2-3. A 3.5-month-old girl with a superficial and deep, segmental hemangioma in the "beard" distribution, at high risk for airway involvement. Note the healing ulceration on the lower lip.

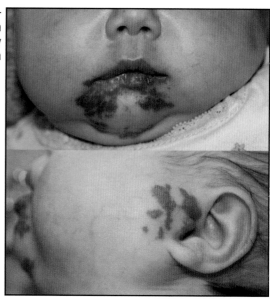

"Beard Area" Hemangiomas

Segmental hemangiomas in the "beard area" (the preauricular/mandibular, lower lip, chin, and neck skin; Figure 2-3) have up to a 60% risk of having symptomatic airway disease. The risk increases if hemangiomas are bilateral and involve more extensive areas of the skin including the neck. Airway hemangiomas often present with inspiratory and expiratory stridor between weeks 4 and 12 of life and are often mistakenly diagnosed as tracheomalacia, upper respiratory infection, or croup. If the hemangioma continues to enlarge, respiratory distress can become life threatening. Even if the hemangioma is only partially occlusive, a superimposed respiratory infection can quickly push the child into respiratory distress. Infants with suspected airway disease should be evaluated promptly by a pediatric otolaryngologist, and if airway disease is present, the patient should be treated aggressively with medical therapies. Hemangiomas involving the parotid gland may require treatment because they can become massive, causing deformity of the ear, cheek, and nose, and, in rare cases, high-output congestive heart failure.

PHACE Syndrome

Patients with facial segmental IHs have a high risk of having a neurocutaneous syndrome known as PHACE, an acronym referring to its variable features including **p**osterior fossa brain malformations, segmental cervicofacial **h**emangioma, **a**rterial anomalies, **c**ardiac defects or coarctation of the aorta, and **e**ye anomalies. Patients with PHACE syndrome may also have sternal defects, such as sternal scars, clefting, or supraumbilical raphe. Up to one-third of patients with large (over 5 cm) segmental facial hemangiomas will be found to have PHACE when studied thoroughly. In all infants with large segmental hemangiomas of the face, consider referral to pediatric dermatology, echocardiogram, magnetic resonance imaging (MRI) and magnetic resonance angiography (MRA) of the head and neck, and formal ophthalmologic examination particularly looking for retinal abnormalities. Periodic developmental and neurologic assessments should be performed.

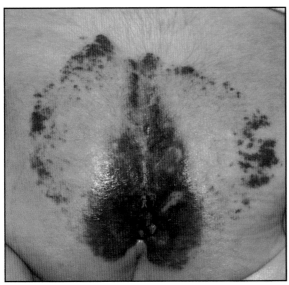

Figure 2-4. Superficial, segmental, lumbosacral IH with perianal ulceration in a 2-month-old girl.

Lumbosacral and Perineal Hemangiomas

Segmental hemangiomas overlying the lumbosacral or perineal area (Figure 2-4) can have associated spinal, bony, and genitourinary anomalies. Several acronyms have been used to describe this association, most recently LUMBAR syndrome (lower body hemangioma and other cutaneous defects, urogenital anomalies, ulceration, myelopathy, bony deformities, anorectal malformations, arterial anomalies, and renal anomalies). Segmental hemangiomas overlying the lumbosacral spine have a significant risk (up to 50%) of spinal dysraphism and tethered spinal cord as well as a risk of intraspinal hemangiomas. MRI is more sensitive than ultrasound for detecting these findings. Renal ultrasound and other investigations should be done based on clinical findings such as abnormal external genitalia.

MULTIFOCAL HEMANGIOMAS

Infants with 5 or more IHs are known to have an increased risk of having hepatic hemangiomas; however, other sites of visceral involvement are extremely rare. Evaluation with liver ultrasound should be considered in infants less than 6 months of age with 5 or more cutaneous hemangiomas.

HEPATIC HEMANGIOMAS

The liver is the most common extracutaneous site of IH. Infants with 5 or more IHs should be evaluated for the possibility of liver hemangiomas with liver ultrasound. Hepatic hemangiomas are often asymptomatic, but in a minority of cases can cause morbidity, and in rare cases are life threatening. High-output cardiac failure can be caused by a few large liver IHs. Abdominal compartment syndrome and hypothyroidism (via tumor-related inactivation of thyroid hormone) can be caused by "diffuse" disease where the liver is virtually replaced by hemangiomas. When there is a large volume or number of IHs, you should check thyroid function tests (thyroid-stimulating hormone [TSH], free

T4, and reverse T3). A high reverse T3 indicates that free T4 is being inactivated by the IH and the thyroid function tests should be followed. Intervention is necessary when a patient with liver IH has cardiac compromise or severe hypothyroidism. Pharmacologic treatment of the IH, aggressive thyroid hormone replacement, embolization, and liver transplant may be considered as therapeutic options.

ULCERATION

Ulceration is the most common complication of IH. Ulceration occurs in approximately 15% of a referral population of patients, usually during the late proliferative phase (4 to 6 months). Segmental, perioral, perianal, and other intertriginous IH (such as the neck) are the most likely to ulcerate (see Figures 2-3 and 2-4). Local wound care and pain control are essential for treatment. Occlusion with either occlusive dressing or thick application of petrolatum-based emollients can help wound healing and decrease the pain of ulceration. Oral acetaminophen with or without hydrocodone and very small amounts of topical lidocaine ointment also help control pain. Ulcerations generally heal with scarring within 2 to 3 weeks with good topical care; however, if these strategies are not successful, you should pursue urgent referral to a pediatric dermatologist or other specialist.

BLEEDING

Many parents are concerned that their child's IHs will "burst" or bleed significantly if it is cut or bumped. With rare exceptions, bleeding is *not* a major problem: hemangiomas are not a "bag of blood," but rather a collection of small blood vessels. Ulcerated IHs sometimes bleed a small amount, but patients with IHs are generally not at risk for a high-pressure, life-threatening bleeding. The exceptions are IHs with deep ulcerations or IHs involving the scalp where everything bleeds more. We tell parents to apply firm, constant pressure to the bleeding area for 15 minutes to get the bleeding to stop.

Suggested Readings

Haggstrom AN, Drolet BA, Baselga E, et al. Prospective study of infantile hemangiomas: clinical characteristics predicting complications and treatment. *Pediatrics.* 2006;118(3):882-887.

Iacobas I, Burrows PE, Frieden IJ, et al. LUMBAR: association between cutaneous infantile hemangiomas of the lower body and regional congenital anomalies. *J Pediatr.* 2010;157(5):795-801, e1-e7.

Kim HJ, Colombo M, Frieden IJ. Ulcerated hemangiomas: clinical characteristics and response to therapy. *J Am Acad Dermatol.* 2001;44(6):962-972.

Metry D, Heyer G, Hess C, et al. Consensus statement on diagnostic criteria for PHACE syndrome. *Pediatrics.* 2009;124(5):1447-1456.

WHAT ARE THE MANAGEMENT/TREATMENT OPTIONS FOR INFANTILE HEMANGIOMAS?

Maria C. Garzon, MD

In order to answer this question, it is essential to take a step back and review the indications for treating infantile hemangiomas (IHs). Not all hemangiomas require active intervention and it is important to remember that there is no single recipe or algorithm for treatment. Management of IH must be individualized. The type of treatment that will be used will depend upon many factors, including the indication for treatment, the presence or absence of systemic associations, the age of the patient, the stage of the hemangioma, and the size and location of the lesion. Many of these factors are interrelated. In most cases, the goal of treatment is to shrink or contain the growth of the IH particularly during the proliferating phase in order to reduce potential complications.

The most common reasons that IH require treatment include the following:
- To prevent or reduce impairment of a vital function
- To improve ulceration, which is often associated with pain and increases the risk of permanent scarring
- To prevent disfigurement (if unchecked growth of the hemangioma will cause distortion that after involution will result in permanent scarring or disfigurement)
- To avoid or treat life-threatening complications (eg, airway compromise)[1,2]

There are also certain morphologic patterns of and anatomic sites at which hemangiomas occur that will help predict whether the patient is at risk for complications (a major factor when selecting therapy). Important patterns include multiple hemangiomas (>5), which are associated with a risk of hepatic hemangiomas (Figure 3-1). Hemangiomas showing a segmental morphology may be associated with systemic involvement including PHACE syndrome (**p**osterior fossa brain malformations, segmental cervicofacial **h**emangioma, **a**rterial anomalies, **c**ardiac defects or **c**oarctation of the aorta, **e**ye anomalies), airway hemangiomas, and what has recently been described as LUMBAR syndrome (**l**ower body hemangioma and other cutaneous defects, **u**rogenital anomalies, **u**lceration, **m**yelopathy, **b**ony deformities, **a**norectal malformations, **a**rterial anomalies, and **r**enal anomalies). Lumbosacral IH is also at high risk for being associated with spinal dysra-

Figure 3-1. Patient with many cutaneous hemangiomas associated with intrahepatic hemangiomas.

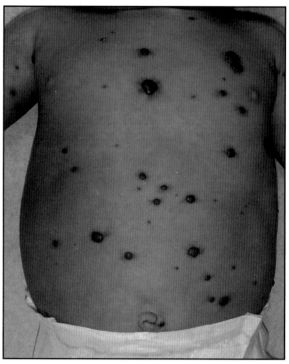

phism including intraspinal extension of the hemangioma. These factors will need to be considered when choosing a management strategy for IH.

Unfortunately, there are few prospective studies that address the management of IH; therefore, much of our knowledge comes from cases series and retrospective reviews. There are no FDA-approved medications for the treatment of IHs and the treatments described in this section represent "off-label use" of drugs approved for other indications and age groups. In this question, I review selected treatment modalities that have been described for the management of IH during the *proliferating* stage of the natural history.

Active Nonintervention

Active nonintervention is a term used to describe a management strategy that includes close periodic monitoring of IH during their life cycle, taking frequent photographs to document growth and involution, and providing families with anticipatory guidance and support regarding the natural history and potential for complications. Hemangiomas are dynamic lesions; therefore, frequent reassessment in the first several months of life is an essential part of this strategy to make sure that a more active treatment is not indicated. Active nonintervention is particularly useful for small, uncomplicated IH with little, if any, risk for leaving a significant residual lesion and is not associated with a risk of functional impairment, disfigurement, or ulceration.

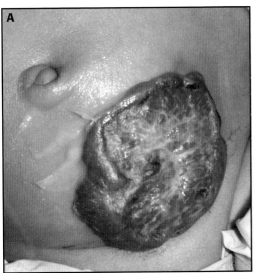 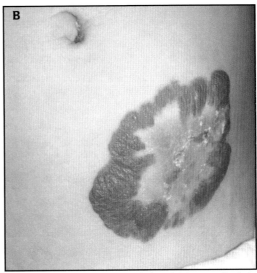

Figure 3-2. (A) Ulcerated hemangioma treated with systemic propranolol, which resulted in (B) rapid healing.

Ulceration/Wound Care

Wound care is often the first-line therapy for ulcerated IH. Ulceration occurs in approximately 10% of IHs[3] often at sites of occlusion/moisture such as the lip, diaper area, or in body folds. However, management of ulcerated IH still must be individualized. For example, the treatment of a severely ulcerated lip or facial hemangioma will differ from that of small area of ulceration within a focal hemangioma in the diaper area, with the more severe ulceration likely to require a systemic medication to control the IH growth (Figure 3-2). Application of topical antibiotics, barrier creams, and nonadherent dressings (eg, petrolatum gauze, hydrocolloid dressings) are frequently used to manage focal ulcerated IHs. A bacterial culture will help assess for secondary bacterial infection. The most commonly used antibiotics include bacitracin and mupirocin. Topical metronidazole use has been reported for hemangiomas in certain locations where anaerobic infections may occur (perianal). In addition, other specialized wound-care dressings and preparations may also have a role in the management of select hemangiomas. Finally, pain management is a cornerstone for the management of ulcerated hemangiomas and consultation with a subspecialist may be indicated.

Topical Therapies

Topical therapies including topical corticosteroids, imiquimod, and most recently topical beta-blockers (specifically topical timolol maleate) have been reported in retrospective case reports for the treatment of IHs. Small IHs that are not causing functional impairment (eg, superficial hemangioma located in a facial location) are often good candidates for topical therapy. The rationale for using a topical treatment would be to spare the infant from the potential side effects of administering a systemic medication. Therefore, the lesions that would be most amenable to this treatment would be small superficial lesions that would provide an easily accessible target and because of size be at low risk for systemic absorption. Clearly widespread application of a topical therapy such as timolol to a large IH or multiple IHs might result in systemic absorption and consequently serious systemic side effects. It is very important to note that some IH may initially appear to be small focal lesions, but in reality they might be "the tip of the iceberg" with a deeper unrecognized portion that has the potential to cause functional impairment (eg, mixed superficial/deep IH in the periocular area). Young infants, especially preterm infants, are at greater risk for systemic absorption of topical medications because of an increased surface area to volume ratio and because of impaired skin barrier function. Finally, the presence of ulceration on the surface of IH may increase the risk of systemic absorption of medications.

Ultrapotent topical corticosteroids have been used to treat superficial hemangiomas with a variable response. Potential side effects include hypopigmentation and atrophy of the surrounding skin and possible systemic absorption.[4] Imiquimod, a topical immune modulator that is approved for the treatment of genital warts and actinic keratoses in adults, is reported to be effective for treating small superficial IH. However, a concern regarding the potential for crusting and superficial ulceration of the IH during treatment has limited its use.[5] Most recently, two authors described their experience using twice daily application of topical timolol maleate 0.5% preparations for smaller superficial hemangiomas. Early reports appear promising but caution is advised because topical timolol applied to intact skin can cause systemic beta blockade.[6,7] In general, all types of topical treatment often need to be continued throughout the proliferating stage in order to prevent rebound growth. Periocular lesions need to be followed by an ophthalmologist for potential adverse reactions and to assure that more aggressive therapy is not required.

Systemic Therapies

The administration of systemic medications to control IH proliferation has been the mainstay of treatment for larger problematic lesions for decades. Systemic prednisolone typically at a dose between 1 and 2 mg/kg/day was often used as the first-line therapy during the proliferating stage. Months of treatment are required. There are multiple potential adverse reactions associated with the long-term use of systemic steroids including adrenal suppression, with infants often becoming cushingoid. Growth delay, immunosuppression, and gastrointestinal (GI) irritability are among other concerning side effects.[8] Coadministration of GI protectants such as ranitidine and more recently pneumocystis prophylaxis has been recommended. Administration of live virus vaccines should be avoided during and for a period following systemic steroid therapy.[9] Recently, it has been noted that the response to immunization may be less protective than desired.[10] Fortunately, when properly monitored most children who received systemic corticosteroids tolerated it without significant long-term sequelae; however, diligent follow-up is essential to manage potential adverse reactions.

A shift in the management of problematic hemangiomas has occurred over the last few years. More recently, oral administration of propranolol at doses between 1 and 2 mg/kg/day divided into 2 or 3 doses/day has been reported to control the growth and shrink proliferating hemangiomas.[11,12] In addition, there appears to be response for some hemangiomas after they have moved out of the phase of most active proliferation after the first year of life.[13] Oral propranolol has also been used to manage problematic ulcerated hemangiomas that are not responsive to more conservative therapy. The optimum dose for ulcerated hemangiomas has not been established. There are no standard protocols regarding the best way to initiate oral propranolol therapy and practices vary considerably. A full discussion of this topic is outside of the scope of this section and recommendations are evolving. Potential adverse reactions including symptomatic hypoglycemia, hypotension, bradycardia, hyperkalemia, and sleep disturbance rebound of growth following cessation of the medication have been described. Baseline cardiac evaluation is recommended with close monitoring. The use of propranolol for problematic hemangiomas needs to be carefully considered and the input of experts with experience using this medication is strongly recommended. Of note, a multicenter, international randomized controlled trial is underway examining the safety and efficacy of this treatment (details at www.clinicaltrials.gov).

The potential for hypotension and bradycardia in patients with PHACE syndrome with significant abnormalities of the cerebrovascular circulation has raised concerns about its use in this population given that some patients with PHACE syndrome are at greater risk for developing strokes. Therefore, it is recommended that infants with large facial hemangiomas (>5 cm in diameter) undergo evaluation for PHACE syndrome before starting oral propranolol so that sufficient information is available to make a decision regarding the treatment in this setting.[14,15]

Pulsed Dye Laser and Excisional Surgery

Pulsed dye lasers (PDLs; wavelength of either 585 or 595 nanometers) have been used to manage ulcerated hemangiomas with reports of healing following a series of treatments to the ulcerated portion. A potential adverse reaction is worsening of the existing ulceration. PDL may also decrease the color and thickness of thin superficial hemangiomas. However, multiple treatments are required during the proliferative phase. Treatment will not halt the proliferation of the deeper component of the IH. Significant ulceration may also complicate PDL treatment. PDL is also used to treat older infants and children with residual telangiectasia on the surface of the hemangioma.

Excisional surgery is most frequently employed to manage residual hemangiomas in locations that are at greatest risk for disfigurement (eg, nasal tip). Many surgeons with expertise in this area favor performing the surgery after the most active phase of proliferation but before 3 to 4 years of age to reduce the psychosocial impact of the residual birthmark. Multiple surgical procedures may be required to achieve a satisfactory result. Early excisional surgery performed by an experienced surgeon during the proliferating stage has been reported and may be used for selected situations including ulcerated lesions amendable to resection, pedunculated lesions, and small focal lesions that are causing functional impairment. There is a risk of rebound growth following surgery since oftentimes only a portion of the hemangioma is removed during surgery.

References

1. Haggstrom AN, Drolet BA, Baselga E, et al. Prospective study of infantile hemangiomas: clinical characteristics predicting complications and treatment. *Pediatrics.* 2006;118(3):882-887.
2. Maguiness SM, Frieden IJ. Current management of infantile hemangiomas. *Semin Cutan Med Surg.* 2010;29(2): 106-114.

3. Chamlin SA, Haggstrom AN, Drolet BA, et al. Multicenter prospective study of ulcerated hemangiomas. *J Pediatr.* 2007;151(6):684-689, 689.e1. Epub 2007 Aug 24.
4. Garzon MC, Lucky AW, Hawrot A, Frieden IJ. Ultrapotent topical corticosteroid treatment of hemangiomas of infancy. *J Am Acad Dermatol.* 2005;52(2):281-286.
5. McCuaig CC, Dubois J, Powell J, et al. A phase II, open-label study of the efficacy and safety of imiquimod in the treatment of superficial and mixed infantile hemangioma. *Pediatr Dermatol.* 2009;26(2):203-312.
6. Guo S, Ni N. Topical treatment for capillary hemangioma of the eyelid using beta-blocker solution. *Arch Ophthalmol.* 2010;128(2):255-256.
7. Pope E, Chakkittakandiyil A. Topical timolol gel for infantile hemangiomas: a pilot study. *Arch Dermatol.* 2010; 146(5):564-565.
8. Bennett ML, Fleischer AB Jr, Chamlin SL, Frieden IJ. Oral corticosteroid use is effective for problematic infantile hemangiomas. An evidence-based evaluation. *Arch Dermatol.* 2001;137(9):1208-2013.
9. Pickering LK, Baker CJ, Kimberlin DW, Long SS, eds. *Red Book: 2009 Report of the Committee on Infectious Diseases.* Elk Grove Village, IL: American Academy of Pediatrics; 2009.
10. Kelly ME, Juern AM, Grossman WJ, Schauer DW, Drolet BA. Immunosuppressive effects in infants treated with corticosteroids for infantile hemangiomas. *Arch Dermatol.* 2010;146(7):767-774.
11. Leaute-Labreze C, Dumas de la Roque E, Hubiche T, Boralevi F, Thambo JB, Taïeb A. Propranolol for severe hemangiomas of infancy. *N Engl J Med.* 2008;358(24):2649-2651.
12. Zvulunov A, McCuaig C, Frieden IJ, et al. Oral propranolol therapy for infantile hemangiomas beyond the proliferation phase: a multicenter retrospective study. *Pediatr Dermatol.* 2011;28(2):94-98. doi: 10.1111/j.1525-1470.2010.01379.x. Epub 2011 March 1.
13. Frieden IJ, Drolet BA. Propranolol for infantile hemangiomas: promise, peril pathogenesis. *Pediatr Dermatol.* 2009;26(5):642-644.
14. Haggstrom AN, Garzon MC, Baselga E, et al. Risk for PHACE syndrome in infants with large facial hemangiomas. *Pediatrics.* 2010;126(2):e418-e426. Epub 2010 Jul 19.
15. Metry DW, Garzon MC, Drolet BA, et al. PHACE syndrome: current knowledge, future directions. *Pediatr Dermatol.* 2009;26(4):381-398.

Suggested Readings

Hong E, Fischer G. Propranolol for the treatment of ulcerated recalcitrant hemangioma of infancy. *Pediatr Dermatol.* 2012;29(1):64-67. Epub 2011 Aug 19.
Saint-Jean M, Léauté-Labrèze C, Mazereeuw-Hautier J, et al. Propranolol for treatment of ulcerated infantile hemangiomas. *J Am Acad Dermatol.* 2011;64(5):827-832. Epub 2011 Feb 25.

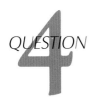

DO ALL SEBACEOUS NEVI NEED TO BE REMOVED?

Magdalene Dohil, MD and Lawrence F. Eichenfield, MD

Nevus sebaceous, also known as nevus sebaceous of Jadassohn, represents a hamartoma or organoid nevus, which is a benign congenital collection of tissue structures. Lesions consist of variable components of the skin organ, including the epidermis, sebaceous glands, hair follicles, apocrine glands, and connective tissue. They are a subtype of an epidermal nevus, which should be included in the differential diagnosis.

It is thought that a nevus sebaceous is due to genetic mosaicism and in some patients the abnormality has been linked to the PTCH gene (the human patched gene), which is also implicated in the evolution of basal cell carcinoma. The cell lines in nevus sebaceous arise from the ectoderm, which develops into the epidermis as well as to neural tissue. This origin explains why lesions may be a cutaneous marker of nevus sebaceous syndrome, usually with a large or dermatomal nevus sebaceous. This syndrome includes ophthalmological, cerebral, and skeletal abnormalities with epileptic seizures being the most common neurological manifestation. Another rare association is that of a nevus sebaceous with a speckled lentiginous nevus, so called phakomatosis pigmentokeratotica, which may present with various neurological problems, hemiatrophy, muscle weakness, and hyperhidrosis.

Most commonly, nevus sebaceous presents at birth as a solitary, initially smooth, yellowish to orange-appearing, hairless plaque with a slightly mammillated surface (Figures 4-1 and 4-2). All races and both sexes are equally affected. Estimated prevalence in newborns in the United States is 0.3%. The most common location is the scalp, but nevus sebaceous may be seen anywhere on the head and neck region. They tend to grow proportionately with the patient and start to show more pronounced changes around adolescence under hormonal stimulation. Clinically this may result in a nevus sebaceous changing into a more bumpy, warty and scaly, greasy growth, causing symptoms of irritation, pruritus, and a cosmetically undesirable hairless bumpy plaque on the scalp.

Later, more commonly in adulthood, other tumors can arise within a nevus sebaceous. These growths vary from benign lesions, such as syringocystadenoma papilliferum, trichoblastoma, and trichilemmoma, to skin cancers including basal cell carcinoma, squamous cell carcinoma, and various skin gland tumors. The exact incidence quoted for

Figure 4-1. A typical alopecic yellow mammillated plaque present at birth on the scalp.

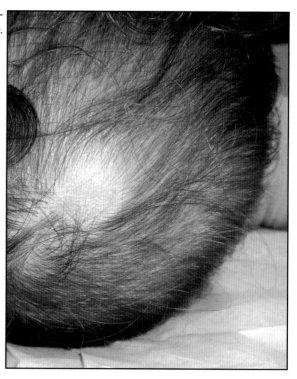

Figure 4-2. Linear yellow nevus sebaceous on the forehead.

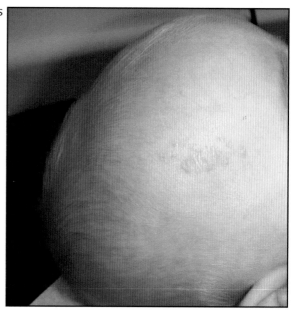

these changes varies greatly and is hard to estimate, since in the past many such lesions were routinely removed during childhood or adolescence. However, the rate of such malignancies is now estimated to be around 1%, far less than was previously estimated at 5% to 22%. Even though they are rare, there are data indicating that both benign and malignant tumors can arise within a nevus sebaceous even in childhood and adolescence.

The differential diagnosis of a nevus sebaceous includes aplasia cutis congenita, epidermal nevus, juvenile xanthogranuloma, and mastocytoma. If the clinical diagnosis is in doubt, a skin biopsy may help to determine the diagnosis prior to considering a more extensive surgical approach, since some of these entities have a tendency toward spontaneous involution.

While prophylactic excision in childhood may not be necessary, our opinion is that elective excision of a nevus sebaceous may be reasonable if the size and location of the lesion favor a cosmetically superior outcome or an apparent clinical change within the lesions makes excision necessary. It is important to engage in a discussion with parents and patients regarding the appropriate timing of the surgery. For many parents, the decision as to when the lesion should be removed is guided by the fear of general anesthesia. Parents should be counseled as to the low risk of anesthesia-related complications when performed electively in a healthy child beyond 6 months of age at a center with extensive pediatric experience. They should also be aware that even in an older child not all sebaceous nevi lend themselves to removal under local anesthesia. Factors that will guide the decision on anesthesia include not only maturity of the child, but also size and location of the lesion, since many scalp lesions tend to bleed profusely and may be approached more safely under the controlled conditions general anesthesia provides. In addition, many facial lesions require complete control of the surgical field and absolute immobilization of the patient to allow for optimal cosmetic outcome. Decision making on small lesions may be deferred until adolescence to allow the patient to be involved in the process with an understanding of the possibility of thickening and benign and malignant growth occurring over a lifetime.

Elective excision during infancy, after the initial neonatal period when the risk for general anesthesia is somewhat higher, may be the appropriate choice for patients where families feel uncomfortable in monitoring the lesion for apparent change over the years and if the hairless area is prominent even at an early age. It is also the option we would recommend for larger lesions, particularly on the scalp, since the pliability of the skin is greater during the first year of life and allows for technically easier primary closure of defects with a lower risk of unwanted spreading of the resulting scar. Postsurgical activity restrictions to support good healing are also much easier to implement in this early age group since the surgery does not interfere with school or sports activities.

Smaller lesions may well be monitored clinically until change is noted within the lesion, which usually occurs during preadolescence. At this time, the patient is often motivated to have the lesion removed due to symptoms of irritation and can be actively involved in the surgical consultation. Many teenage patients will be able to tolerate the surgery under local anesthesia, and they are able to understand their role in successful postsurgical care and activity restrictions. However, spreading of scars appears to have a higher incidence in this age group, since adherence to activity limitations greatly varies and is hard to enforce beyond a 2- to 3-week initial recovery period.

Summary

Nevus sebaceous is a commonly encountered benign birthmark of the scalp and head that, when symptomatic with clinical apparent change over time, is treated by surgical excision. If surgery is being done electively, the timing of surgery is debatable and various concerns need to be taken into consideration. We tell our patients and families that for most lesions, early "prophylactic excision" is no longer recommended, but that excision is reasonable for larger and cosmetically prominent lesions and should be pursued for clinically symptomatic or changing lesions.

Suggested Readings

Jaqueti G, Requena L, Sanchez Yus E. Trichoblastoma is the most common neoplasm developed in nevus sebaceous of Jadassohn; a clinicopathologic study of a series of 155 cases. *Am J Dermatopathol.* 2000;22(2):108-118.

Rosen H, Schmidt B, Lam HP, Meara JG, Labow BI. Management of nevus sebaceous and the risk of basal cell carcinoma: an 18-year review. *Pediatr Dermatol.* 2009;26(6):676-681. Epub 2009 Jul 20.

Santibanez-Gallerani A, Marshall D, Duarte AM, Melnick SJ, Thaller S. Should nevus sebaceus of Jadassohn in children be excised? A study of 757 cases, and literature review. *J Craniofac Surg.* 2003;14(5):658-660.

WHEN DO I WORRY ABOUT
MIDLINE CUTANEOUS LUMBOSACRAL LESIONS?

Christine T. Lauren, MD

It is important to spend a few minutes performing a full skin examination on every new patient in your office. We have made several incidental diagnoses with regard to abnormalities of the lumbosacral area after performing a complete examination.

Spinal dysraphism is defined as a developmental abnormality in the formation of the spinal cord or its associated surrounding midline structures. Open spinal dysraphism, or spina bifida aperta, refers to an abnormality with exposed neural tissue, such as is seen in a myelomeningocele. It is referred to as occult spinal dysraphism, or spina bifida occulta, when the spinal abnormality is covered without visible connection to the cutaneous surface. Intraspinal findings associated with occult spinal dysraphism include fatty accumulations (lipomyelomeningocele, spinal lipoma, and fatty filum), dermal sinus, or diastematomyelia (split cord). *Tethered cord* is a term used to describe when the (normally freely mobile) distal spinal cord is abnormally attached to surrounding structures. Over a lifetime, these abnormalities can lead to irreversible neurologic damage. Early diagnosis, serial monitoring, and surgical intervention, if indicated, can improve overall prognosis. Many times, there will be a cutaneous marker overlying a patient's spinal abnormality. Your role as the pediatrician or dermatologist is to correctly identify the cutaneous lesion, classify its associated risk of occult spinal dysraphism, and refer for screening evaluation of an underlying abnormality when appropriate.

Examination of the lumbosacral area is best performed with the child in the prone position. Inspect for any visible midline lumbosacral cutaneous lesions as well as palpate for deeper subcutaneous anomalies not appreciable with inspection alone. Apply lateral pressure to the buttocks to fully examine the symmetry of the gluteal cleft as well as its base for any dimpling or pitting. Measure the distance between the cutaneous lesion and the anal verge. Examine the perineum for any anogenital anomalies.

We have learned that a combination of two or more cutaneous features place the patient at highest risk of occult spinal dysraphism; examples might include a subcutaneous lipoma with an overlying vascular stain or an area of hypertrichosis with an associated atypical

Figure 5-1. Large melanocytic nevus over the upper lumbosacral spine with hypertrichosis and associated atypical ventriculus terminalis found on MRI.

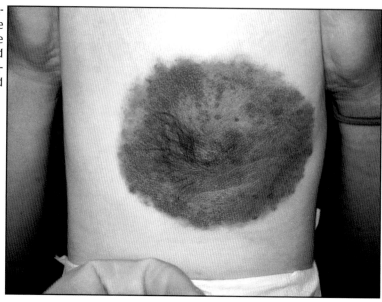

dimple. Such lesions require radiographic screening. In addition, cutaneous anorectal abnormalities have been found to correlate highly with underlying spinal dysraphism. Midline lumbosacral lipomas, which may be superficial or penetrate deeply, are strong markers for associated spinal anomalies. Melanocytic nevi on the lumbosacral area can be associated with spinal dysraphism as well as neurocutaneous melanosis (Figure 5-1). Other lesions that warrant further evaluation include a midline or paramedian area of aplasia cutis or a "pseudo-tail" (acrochordon or skin tag). Hypertrichosis localized to the lumbosacral spine, alone or in association with additional cutaneous anomalies, warrants a thorough evaluation. The term *faun tail* is used to describe a focal area of long coarse or silky hair that is often V-shaped in distribution. More subtle hair excess may be a normal variant in the lumbosacral region.

A recent study by Drolet et al highlights the strong association of a cutaneous lumbosacral hemangioma and underlying spinal dysraphism (Figure 5-2). Approximately one in three patients with an isolated midline sacral hemangioma was found to have associated intraspinal anomalies, most commonly an intraspinal lipoma or intraspinal hemangioma. This risk increased further if the hemangioma was found in association with one or more additional cutaneous abnormalities. Of note, an ulcer in the perineum of an infant (as in Figure 5-2) may be the first cutaneous sign of a hemangioma.

The term *nevus simplex* to the physician refers to the near ubiquitous findings on neonatal examination of an eyelid "angel's kiss" or nape of neck "stork bite." A recent study by Juern et al highlights the midline lumbosacral area as a not uncommon site of nevus simplex. Controversy exists in the literature as to the utility of screening these patients for occult spinal dysraphism. A sacral vascular patch in a neonate/infant with associated nevus simplex elsewhere (eyelid, glabella, forehead, nape of neck) may be serially monitored. An isolated midline sacral stain should be observed for lightening with anticipatory guidance given regarding developmental warning signs. If noted in childhood or young adulthood, a vascular stain may represent a true capillary malformation or "port wine stain"; as in the majority of cases of nevus simplex, the lesion fades

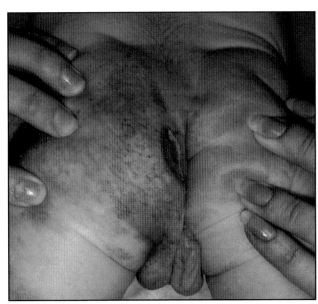

Figure 5-2. Large segmental hemangioma over the lumbosacral spine with an associated lipomyelomeningocele and spinal cord tethering.

over time. Although not generally considered a "high-risk" lesion, discussion of the reported association of an isolated capillary malformation with spinal anomalies should take place with a patient's family and their primary care physician. Decision to image should be individualized in these cases. In association with a second cutaneous marker, a vascular stain does warrant an evaluation for spinal dysraphism.

A sacral dimple is one of the most common cutaneous abnormalities identified on lumbosacral skin examination. A typical or simple dimple is a lesion greater than 5 mm in diameter, located in the midline of the gluteal cleft, shallow with a visible base and originates less than 2.5 cm from the anal verge. Also referred to as a coccygeal pit, these lesions are not considered markers of occult spinal dysraphism. On the other hand, an atypical dimple is a strong predictor of underlying dysraphism. Atypical dimples include those originating greater than 2.5 cm from the anal verge, off-midline in position, or wider than 5 mm in diameter. Along with gluteal crease asymmetry, these lesions may indicate an underlying dermal sinus tract or other spinal anomaly. These tracts extend from the skin surface and may communicate with the central nervous system. This communication places the patient not only at an infection risk but also at risk for tethering of the spinal cord.

Obtaining a focused review of systems and targeted examination is time well spent as these symptoms have been appreciated in many children with tethered spinal cord. Elicit associated signs such as bowel or bladder habit changes or any notable change in motor skill set. Ask older children about lower extremity pain, numbness, or weakness. General examination should make note of any lower extremity discrepancies in size, bulk, strength or reflexes. These findings are present when there are in fact neurologic sequelae present. We strive to identify those asymptomatic children who, based on a cutaneous sign, may be at risk for future neurologic decline if untreated.

The best screening tool for spinal dysraphism depends on the individual patient, his or her age, and the lesion in question. Ultrasound of the lumbosacral spine is a cost-effective examination that poses no associated risk of sedation or risk assumed from the procedure itself. However, by 5 to 6 months of age or earlier in some cases, bony structures calcify, making this technology inadequate. Ultrasound may not have the adequate resolution needed to detect a small sinus tract. Thick cutaneous or subcutaneous lesions may make satisfactory evaluation of the underlying spine by ultrasound difficult. There are documented reports of negative ultrasound studies with subsequent anomalies demonstrated on magnetic resonance imaging (MRI). Should an ultrasound demonstrate an abnormality, a follow-up MRI should be obtained to better delineate the anatomic defect. MRI is the screening examination of choice in our practice in the older infant and in a child with a high-risk lesion; a negative MRI can more definitively eliminate the risk of spinal dysraphism for a family.

Timing of radiographic screening is also a topic of some debate. Vascular lesions such as hemangiomas have a predictable natural history. Intraspinal lesions, like their cutaneous counterparts, may not be present at birth or as appreciable in the first few months of life. Performing a screening examination of the spine too early, whether ultrasound or MRI, may miss a proliferating lesion such as a hemangioma. We will often defer more invasive imaging such as an MRI until a child is a few months of age, so that the likelihood of a false negative is lower. Noninvasive ultrasonography may be repeated at intervals to assure that a vascular lesion has not manifested itself to a level detectable on serial imaging.

Consultation with pediatric neurosurgery is indicated should an abnormality be identified so that a full discussion of the anticipated natural history of the lesion may be performed. In addition, indications to treat may be discussed along with the associated risks, benefits, and timing of therapy. Neurologic or neurosurgical consultation may also be helpful with a borderline cutaneous lesion, when imaging is contraindicated or considered high risk, or should a parent have reservations about the sedation risks associated with imaging.

Suggested Readings

Drolet B. Cutaneous signs of neural tube malformations. *Semin Cutan Med Surg.* 2004;23(2):125-137.

Drolet BA, Chamlin SL, Garzon MC, et al. Prospective study of spinal anomalies in children with infantile hemangiomas of the lumbosacral skin. *J Pediatr.* 2010;157(5):789-794. Epub 2010 Sep 9.

Guggisberg D, Hadj-Rabia S, Viney C, et al. Skin markers of occult spinal dysraphism in children: a review of 54 cases. *Arch Dermatol.* 2004;140(9):1109-1115.

Juern AM, Glick ZR, Drolet BA, Frieden IJ. Nevus simplex: a reconsideration of nomenclature, sites of involvement, and disease associations. *J Am Acad Dermatol.* 2010;63(5):805-814. Epub 2010 Aug 21.

Sardana K, Gupta R, Garg VK, et al. A prospective study of cutaneous manifestations of spinal dysraphism from India. *Pediatr Dermatol.* 2009;26(6):688-695.

QUESTION

6

HOW DO I EVALUATE WHITE BIRTHMARKS?

Anna S. Salinas, MD and Moise L. Levy, MD

As with any possible birthmark, the evaluation of a white skin lesion should begin by seeking the answers to a few key questions (Table 6-1).

1. What is the age of the patient, and how long has the mark been present? In other words is it truly a "birthmark" (congenital) or, in an older child, is there a possibility that the mark has recently appeared (acquired)?
2. Where on the body is the mark located?
3. What is the size of the mark?
4. Is the mark truly depigmented (stark white), or is it hypopigmented (lighter in color than the surrounding skin but not completely white)?
5. Has the mark changed from its original appearance?
6. Are there other marks present on the child's body? If so, is there any sort of pattern to the lesions?
7. Are there symptoms such as pruritus? Is there scaling present? Is the area anesthetic?
8. When considering genodermatoses: Does the child manifest any other dermatologic or systemic findings?

After the answers to these questions have been determined, you may begin to divide the likely etiology of the lesion into one of the following broad categories:

- *Congenital birthmarks* including the most common white birthmark, nevus depigmentosus (seen in 1/130 healthy infants) as well as hypomelanosis of Ito or incontinentia pigmenti achromians (if with neurodevelopmental features), halo nevus (depigmentation around a mole, not usually congenital), and nevus anemicus.
- *Acquired hypo- or depigmented macules or patches* such as those secondary to infectious, inflammatory, or traumatic etiologies, including vitiligo, postinflammatory hypopigmentation, pityriasis alba, lichen sclerosis, tinea versicolor, and leprosy.
- *Congenital manifestations of birthmarks* including piebaldism, Waardenburg syndrome, and tuberous sclerosis.

Table 6-1

Differential Diagnosis of White Skin Lesions

	Age of Patient When Mark Manifests	Location on Body	Size/ Shape/ Pattern	Depigmented or Hypopigmented	Changing Morphology	Associated Findings	Key Pieces of History/Physical
Nevus depigmentosus (Figure 6-1)	92% present by 3 years of age	Back and buttocks most common, followed by chest, abdomen, neck, and arms	Isolated type: Circumscribed, small, and round with serrated borders Segmental type: Often over 10 cm and present in linear fashion	Often hypopigmented, rarely depigmented	No—mark tends to be stable	Solitary or multiple; can be segmental	Highlighted with Wood lamp
Hypomelanosis of Ito (Incontinentia pigmenti achromians)	At birth or acquired in first year of life	Trunk, extremities (spares palms, soles, mucous membranes)	Whorled, linear—follows lines of Blaschko	Hypopigmented	May fade in adulthood	Usually multiple and segmental (or mosaic)	Associated neurologic, ocular, and/or skeletal abnormalities (limb hemihypertrophy) present in up to 60% of patients
Halo nevus (see Figure 10-4) (Sutton nevus, perinevoid vitiligo)	Usually acquired; can be congenital, occurring around a melanocytic nevus	Random	The white ring is typically uniform around the nevus	Depigmented	Depigmentation around original pigmented nevus; original nevus may disappear; may repigment or depigmentation may remain	This can be a premonitory sign of vitiligo	Consider melanoma by evaluating the residual mole in older children with family history of melanoma

(continued)

Table 6-1 (continued)

Differential Diagnosis of White Skin Lesions

	Age of Patient When Mark Manifests	Location on Body	Size/ Shape/ Pattern	Depigmented or Hypopigmented	Changing Morphology	Associated Findings	Key Pieces of History/Physical
Ash leaf spots/ macules (Figure 6-2)	Present at birth	Torso/elsewhere	Sharply demarcated pale macules or patches	Hypopigmented	No	May be multiple	Consider tuberous sclerosis if 3 or more, see Table 6-2 (however, 2 to 3/1000 normal newborns have an ash leaf spot)
Nevus anemicus (Figure 6-3)	At birth or acquired in first year of life	Anywhere	1 to 3 cm in diameter, round with irregular borders	Hypopigmented	No	Rarely associated with other birthmarks	If pressure is applied with a convex glass, the lesion disappears (diascopy). If stroked, no flare is elicited
Vitiligo	Rare in infancy, more common in childhood	Anywhere; often periorificial, elbows, knees, ankles, or other frictional areas	Macules, patches, segmental	Hypopigmented (early) then depigmented	Not usually unless repigmenting or extending	No	Chalky white when examined under Wood lamp
Postinflammatory hypopigmentation	Any age	Anywhere	Dependent upon preceding pattern of inflammation or injury	Depigmented or hypopigmented	May regress with time	Often multiple	History of inflammation or injury
Pityriasis alba (many consider to be a subset of postinflammatory hypopigmentation)	More common in childhood than in infancy	Face more often than extremities— light	Usually round	Hypopigmentation	May develop fine scale	No	Child may have history of atopic disease

(continued)

Table 6-1 (continued)

Differential Diagnosis of White Skin Lesions

	Age of Patient When Mark Manifests	Location on Body	Size/ Shape/ Pattern	Depigmented or Hypopigmented	Changing Morphology	Associated Findings	Key Pieces of History/Physical
Lichen sclerosus	Any age, though uncommon in infants	Typically in genital or perianal area can be extragenital	"Figure 21-1" distribution on anogenital skin (female)	Depigmented	May have atrophy or sclerosis	Erythema, vesiculation xerosis	Burning, pruritic More common in females May present with dysuria or constipation
Lichen striatus	More common in children and adolescents, rare in infants	Extremities, facial, truncal	Linear papular and dermatitic early; follows lines of Blaschko	Hypopigmented	Resolves over years with ultimate repigmentation	Rarely involves the nail as well	Thin line that progresses from popular to flat hypopigmented over months
Pityriasis/tinea versicolor	Any age, more common in puberty	Often face, upper torso, shoulders	Round, may coalesce	Hypopigmented; may be hyperpigmented on dark skin	With scale	Severe, widespread Tinea versicolor can be seen in pregnancy and immunodeficient states such as HIV infection	Pruritic, spores, and hyphae "spaghetti and meatballs" by microscopic examination (KOH)
Leprosy/Hansen disease	Any age, though not congenital	Anywhere	May follow dermatomes	Hypopigmented	Individual lesions often slowly enlarge	There will often be multiple spots	The hypopigmented area may be anesthetic

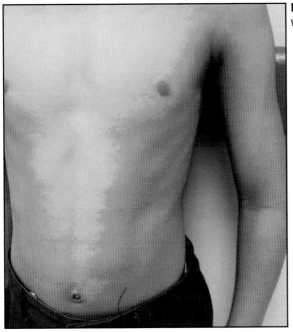

Figure 6-1. Isolated hypopigmented patch with midline cutoff on this healthy patient.

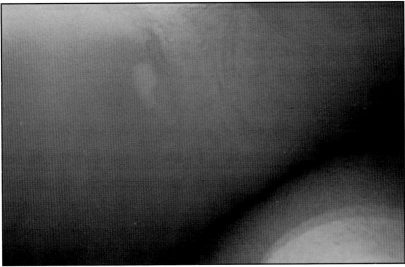

Figure 6-2. Small ash leaf macule on the left flank.

Figure 6-3. Nevus anemicus on the right upper chest.

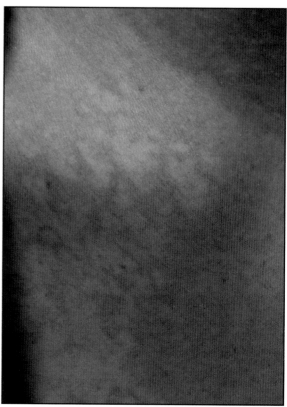

Within these broad categories, a white skin lesion may be differentiated by its appearance and natural history.

A Wood lamp may be helpful to identify areas of hypo- or depigmentation in light-skinned patients. Depigmented areas will highlight dramatically with Wood light and subtle areas of hypopigmentation may become apparent. This is an extremely useful tool when trying to count the number of ash leaf macules in a patient to determine the risk of tuberous sclerosis, for instance.

In some cases, a skin biopsy with subsequent histologic analysis might be necessary to distinguish the various lesions such as leprosy and lichen sclerosis.

The key characteristics that differentiate "white marks" can be found in Table 6-1. Using clinical history, signs, and symptoms, white marks are often readily distinguishable. Finally, a brief outline of the key findings of the genodermatoses that manifest with "white marks" is provided in Table 6-2.

Table 6-2
Genodermatoses With Hypopigmentation

	Lesion Description	*Location of Lesions*	*Change*	*Associated Findings*
Piebaldism autosomal dominant (AD)	Depigmented patches with hyperpigmented borders, often symmetric	Forehead, neck, anterior trunk, anterior legs	Grow proportionally with child, but do not progress	Family history of piebaldism, white forelock
Tuberous sclerosis (AD)	Polygonal, lance-ovate ("ash leaf spot"), and guttate macules. Usually more than 3 lesions present at birth	Anywhere	No, however a Wood light may be helpful in identifying subtle lesions	Angiofibromas, seizures, mental retardation, connective tissue nevi, periungual fibroma. High rate of new mutations
Waardenburg syndrome (types 1 to 4) (AD)	Patchy depigmentation of the hair and skin	Scalp and trunk	Grow proportionally with child but do not progress	Abnormalities of vision, hearing, facial dysmorphia (lateral displacement of inner canthi, broad nasal root), white forelock

Suggested Readings

Conlon JD, Drolet BA. Skin lesions in the neonate. *Pediatr Clin North Am.* 2004;51(4):863-868, vii-viii.

Dohil MA, Baugh WP, Eichenfield LF. Vascular and pigmented birthmarks. *Pediatr Clin North Am.* 2000;47(4): 738-812, v-vi.

Happle, R. Mosaicism in human skin. *Arch Dermatol.* 1993;129(11): 1460-1470.

Lee HS, Chun YS, Hann SK. Nevus depigmentosus: clinical features and histopathologic characteristics in 67 patients. *J Am Acad Dermatol.* 1999;40(1):21-26.

Ruiz-Maldonado, R. Hypomelanotic conditions of the newborn and infant. *Dermatol Clin.* 2007;25(3):373-382, ix.

How Do I Evaluate Tan Birthmarks?

Patrick McMahon, MD

The vast majority of tan birthmarks are inconsequential; however, there are certain physical examination features that can alert a physician to the possibility of an underlying genetic syndrome or systemic disease. For the purpose of this review, the term *birthmark* will include those lesions noted at *or* soon after birth, as some pigmented birthmarks can be present, but are less noticeable, at the time of birth. In this review, I will outline a quick approach to tan birthmarks that can be utilized during the newborn physical examination. Specifically, your evaluation should focus on the size, number, and distribution of these birthmarks. As always, such an evaluation should include a full skin and mucous membrane examination and a thorough evaluation of the child's global development.[1]

Solitary Tan Birthmarks

Generally speaking, solitary tan birthmarks are of little concern and reassurance can be provided. This is especially true for small (<5 mm) birthmarks, which usually represent benign lesions, such as a café-au-lait macule (CALM; Figure 7-1), a lightly pigmented congenital melanocytic nevus, a solitary mastocytoma, or a juvenile xanthogranuloma (JXG). Mastocytomas often appear in the first 3 months of life as flesh-colored or light brown macules, papules, or nodules. Upon stroking of a mastocytoma, it may demonstrate an urticarial appearance secondary to release of histamine from its mast cells, a clinical clue known as Darier sign. JXGs are firm, well-defined yellow, brown, or pink papules or nodules. In 20% of cases, JXGs are present at birth while the remainder usually present later in infancy.[2] Upon compression with a glass slide, a maneuver known as diascopy, a yellowish color can be appreciated that can be a clue to this diagnosis. For all of the aforementioned solitary birthmarks, if they remain stable in size and shape and there are no other birthmarks, clinical monitoring is sufficient.

In larger (>5 mm) solitary birthmarks, distribution and shape become important. In most cases, the patient simply has a larger isolated CALM. If you encounter a patient with a very large (usually several centimeters) block-like CALM, located on one-half of a newborn's trunk, this likely represents a condition that has been termed *segmental pigmentation disorder* (Figure 7-2). An isolated lesion is unlikely to be associated with

Figure 7-1. Café-au-lait macules on the back.

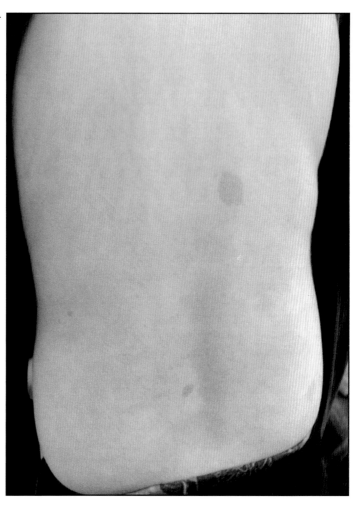

Figure 7-2. Segmental pigmentary disorder in a developmentally normal patient.

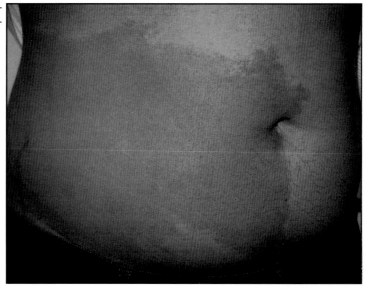

extracutaneous findings and this patient can be monitored clinically for normal growth and development.[3] Similarly, a linear or swirled pigmented birthmark is often a sign of pigmentary mosaicism. This umbrella term includes conditions wherein relatively darker (hyperpigmented) or lighter (hypopigmented) skin is found in a linear distribution, following the so-called *lines of Blaschko*. These unusually shaped lines are thought to represent embryonal migration patterns within the skin. They appear as linear streaks on the arms and legs, often wrapping from posterior to anterior, S-shaped on the chest and V-shaped on the back.[1] The term *nevoid hypermelanosis* has been used to describe the subset of patients with hyperpigmented birthmarks that are found in this distribution. Isolated lesions of nevoid hypermelanosis can be managed with reassurance and clinical monitoring, as extracutaneous anomalies are exceedingly rare. If the birthmark is persistent past infancy, darkening, and in an anatomically sensitive location, such as the face, referral to a specialist would be reasonable. Lastly, in approaching a female patient with a linear birthmark that appears to represent mosaicism, it is important to incontinentia pigmenti (IP). This X-linked dominant condition presents at or soon after birth with lesions following the lines of Blaschko that progress from blisters to verrucous papules. Pigment deposition in the dermis can subsequently manifest as linear brown streaks. For this reason, in a female neonate with linear hyperpigmentation, I recommend simply questioning the caretaker if the "birthmark" was preceded by a vesicular or papular streak. If IP is suspected, referral to a pediatric dermatologist is warranted for further evaluation.

Multiple Tan Birthmarks

A patient with multiple tan birthmarks requires a careful physical examination and will often need to be referred to pediatric dermatology and/or genetics to be evaluated. If you are presented with a newborn who has several small (<5 mm) well-defined tan-to-light brown macules, these may represent multiple lentigines. Depending on their location, these may be a sign of an underlying systemic condition (Table 7-1) and, therefore, they should prompt a referral to a specialist.

Evaluating a patient with multiple CALMs requires precise documentation of size and number to screen for an associated disorder, namely neurofibromatosis-1 (NF-1). As a criterion for NF-1, a patient must have 6 or greater CALMs, each greater than 5 mm. If a patient meets this criterion, direct referral to genetics and/or pediatric dermatology is needed to evaluate him or her for any other evidence of NF-1. If the above criterion is not met, but the patient has several CALMs, I would advocate for serial examinations since other suggestive physical examination findings may develop in the first few years of life. These findings include axillary or inguinal freckling, neurofibromas, or relative macrocephaly. Of note, in some patients with NF-1, a plexiform neurofibroma may be present at birth. These plexiform neurofibromas may appear as brown-red plaques and can have a soft baggy feel upon palpation. Furthermore, a family history of NF-1 should be explored as it is inherited in an autosomal dominant fashion. Multiple large CALMs can be associated with several other syndromes (Table 7-2). For this reason, referring such patients to a specialist is reasonable.

Table 7-1

Multiple Lentigines

Condition	Location of Lesions	Associated Findings
LEOPARD syndrome	Widespread on face, neck, upper trunk, upper arms, spares mucous membranes	**L**entigines **E**lectrocardiographic conduction defects **O**cular hypertelorism **P**ulmonary stenosis **A**bnormalities of genitalia **R**etardation of growth **D**eafness (sensorineural)
Carney complex (includes NAME and LAMB syndrome)	Central face > neck, trunk, extremities, and genitalia Can involve mucous membranes	**N**evi **A**trial myxoma **M**yxoid neurofibroma **E**phelides (aka freckles) **L**entigines **A**trial myxoma **M**yxoid tumors **B**lue nevi Carney complex is also associated with testicular Sertoli tumors, pituitary adenomas (acromegaly), psammomatous melanotic Schwannomas
Peutz-Jeghers syndrome	Lips, buccal mucosa > palate, gingiva, face, fingers, elbows, palms, toes > periumbilical, perianal, labial	Gastrointestinal polyps Slight increased risk of gastrointestinal and other malignancies later in life
Bannayan-Riley-Ruvalcaba syndrome	Penile shaft or vulva	Macrocepahly Multiple subcutaneous and/or visceral lipomas Vascular malformations Intestinal polyps
Zosteriform lentiginous nevus (nevus spilus)	Segmentally distributed macules within a larger tan patch. Usually unilateral	Rare cases of melanoma reported[4]
Segmental lentiginosis	Clustered macules on a background of normal skin	Reports of ipsilateral cerebrovascular hypertrophy and proliferation, pes cavus, and prominent neuropsychiatric findings[5]
Inherited patterned lentiginosis	Facial, lip, extremity, buttock, palmoplantar	Benign, reported in lightly pigmented African Americans[6]

Table 7-2
Multiple Café-Au-Lait Macules

Condition	Associated Findings
Familial Inherited CALM	No systemic abnormalities
NF-1	Neurofibromas Axillary/inguinal freckling Optic glioma Lisch nodules (iris hamartoma) Bone changes (sphenoid wing dysplasia or pseudoarthrosis)[1]
Neurofibromatosis type 2	Bilateral schwannomas, meningiomas, and spinal tumors
McCune-Albright syndrome	Polyostotic fibrous dysplasia Multiple endocrine abnormalities (precocious puberty, hyperthyroidism, Cushing syndrome, etc)
Segmental pigmentation disorder	Rare systemic abnormalities[3]
Legius syndrome	NF-like features Intertriginous freckling Lipomas Macrocephaly Developmental delays[7]
Watson syndrome	Intertriginous freckling Short stature Pulmonary stenosis Low intelligence[1]
Ring chromosome syndrome	Hemangiomas Nevus flammeus (salmon patch) Congenital melanocytic nevi

CALM indicates café-au-lait macules

Figure 7-3. Lines of postinflammatory hyperpigmentation related to skin folding in utero that resolved on their own.

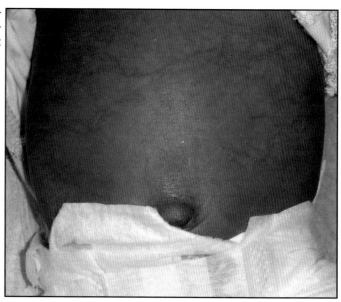

In the case of a patient with multiple linear or whorled tan or brown birthmarks (see previous discussion), referral would also be warranted due to the possibility of an associated syndrome. These include epidermal nevus syndrome, phakomatosis pigmentovascularis, IP, or nevoid hypermelanosis with or without anomalies. This should not be confused with hyperpigmentation from skin wrinkling in utero, which will fade spontaneously (Figure 7-3).

If there are multiple lesions that are consistent with mastocytomas or JXGs as discussed above, then referral to a dermatologist would be prudent to assess appropriately for evidence of extracutaneous manifestations and treat accordingly.

Summary

Isolated tan birthmarks of any size are uniformly less likely to be associated with an underlying condition. Conversely, having multiple tan birthmarks can be a harbinger of an underlying genetic syndrome and more often warrants referral. The distribution of these birthmarks can at times be an interesting clue to an underlying pattern of pigmentary mosaicism, which in isolation is of little concern. In all cases, a full physical examination and serial monitoring are essential in order to screen for any further evidence of a systemic condition.

References

1. Gibbs NF, Makkar H. Disorders of hyperpigmentation and melanocytes. In: Eichenfield, LF, Frieden, IJ, Esterly, NB. *Neonatal Dermatology*. 2nd ed. Philadelphia, PA: Saunders Elsevier, 2008.
2. Paller, AS, Mancini AJ. *Hurwitz Clinical Pediatric Dermatology: A Textbook of Skin Disorders of Childhood and Adolescence*. 3rd ed. Philadelphia, PA: Elsevier Saunders; 2006.
3. Treat J. Patterned pigmentation in children. *Pediatr Clin North Am*. 2010;57(5):1121-1129.
4. Bolognia JL. Fatal melanoma arising in a zosteriform speckled lentiginous nevus. *Arch Dermatol*. 1991;127(8): 1240-1241.
5. Trattner A, Metzker A. Partial unilateral lentiginosis. *J Am Acad Dermatol*. 1993;29(5 Pt 1):693-695.
6. O'Neill J, James WD. Inherited patterned lentiginosis in blacks. *Arch Dermatol*. 1989;125(9):1231-1235.
7. Stevenson D, Viskochil D, Mao R, Muram-Zborovski T. Legius syndrome. 2010 October. In: Pagon RA, Bird TC, Dolan CR, Stephens K, eds. *GeneReviews* [Internet]. Seattle, WA: University of Washington, Seattle; 1993.

WHAT DO I NEED TO CONSIDER DIAGNOSTICALLY AND THERAPEUTICALLY WITH FACIAL PORT-WINE STAINS?

Magdalene Dohil, MD and Lawrence F. Eichenfield, MD

Port-Wine Stains

Port-wine stains (PWS) are vascular capillary malformations that are usually present at birth. The estimated incidence is about 0.3% of newborns. Lesions appear as macular blotches of pink, red, or purple skin on any part of the body. Although congenital, they may continue to evolve and become more noticeable over time. While most PWS occur without other anomalies, they may also occur as part of other malformations, including venous, lymphatic, arteriovenous, or combinations of vessel type. In addition, PWS are part of the presenting findings for several syndromes, including Sturge-Weber syndrome (SWS) and Klippel-Trenaunay syndrome (see next), and may be part of more complex vascular malformations. Most lesions occur sporadically, but there are rare families with multiple PWS diffusely distributed over the body, in which an autosomal dominant pattern of inheritance has been observed.

Cutaneous Findings

At birth, PWS present as flat patches of various size, usually on one side of the body and often in a dermatomal distribution, often with a midline cut-off (Figure 8-1). The face tends to be commonly affected. PWS grow proportionately, and if left untreated, do not resolve.

Often they are felt to lighten over the first 3 to 6 months of life, but this phenomenon is due to the decrease in blood hemoglobin concentration (typically 15 to 17 g/dL at birth to a nadir of 8 to 10 g/dL by age 3 months) and does not indicate true resolution. Rather

Figure 8-1. PWS in a V3 distribution on the right face of this infant.

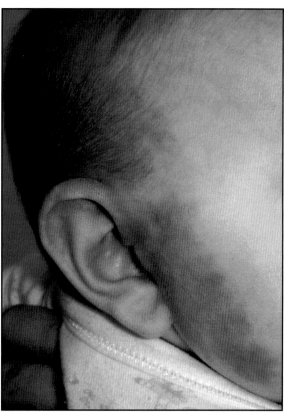

the natural evolution of PWS over a lifetime is marked by gradual darkening from pink-red to a crimson or deep purple with possible associated skin thickening, soft tissue hypertrophy, and vascular blebs that may result in functional compromise and cosmetic disfigurement. This may be seen in particular with facial PWS in the distribution of the second branch of the trigeminal nerve (V2 distributed) PWS. Eczematous changes within a PWS are also not uncommon.

PWS may be associated with other congenital birthmarks. The association of PWS ("nevus flammeus") with pigmentary anomalies, such as extensive mongolian spots, nevus spilus, or nevoid hyperpigmentation, is a feature of phakomatosis pigmentovascularis. Recently an autosomal dominant PWS syndrome caused by RASA-1 mutation has been identified. Patients often have multiple PWS, a positive family history, and are at risk for arteriovenous malformations (AVMs), including in the central nervous system. Genetic testing is readily available and these patients may require further work-up to rule out AVMs.

Management and Treatment

Given the tendency to gradual thickening and nodularity of PWS, treatment is indicated, generally early in life. Treatment is often advised during infancy and childhood as clinical data indicate a tendency for better treatment response and prevention of progressive

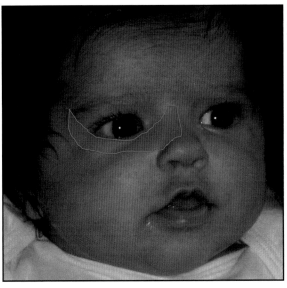

Figure 8-2. The purple area of color denotes the potential overlap of V1 and V2 in this healthy infant.

change over time. Early treatment also helps to minimize possible stigmatization of the child, as the necessary treatment course may be completed prior to preschool entry.

The flashlamp-pumped pulsed dye laser (FPDL) is a universally established treatment modality for PWS with a very low risk of scarring, even in young infants. About 10% to 15% of PWS are reported to clear completely with FPDL, whereas the majority of treated lesions lighten significantly. Response to laser treatment varies by facial region: the face and neck improve more promptly, though less so in the V2 distribution than other facial sites. Advanced laser technology, including epidermal cooling devices, have allowed more effective treatment, even in darker-skinned individuals. Patients and families should, however, be made aware of the risk of "redarkening" of a previously treated stain over time.

Special attention should be paid to the diagnosis and work-up of certain facial PWS, which may be associated with SWS, also known as encephalotrigeminal angiomatosis. The syndrome describes the association of a capillary vascular malformation affecting the skin supplied by one branch of the trigeminal nerve of the face with defects in the underlying tissues.

The classic triad in SWS includes the association of a facial PWS involving the first batch of the trigeminal nerve (V1-ophthalmic), although it may extend beyond this area, ipsilateral eye abnormalities (choroidal vascular anomalies, increased ocular pressure, buphthalmos, and glaucoma in about 30%), and leptomeningeal and brain abnormalities (leptomeningeal vascular malformation, calcifications, cerebral atrophy, enlarged choroid plexus, and developmental venous anomalies in the brain).

The risk of SWS with a V1 PWS alone is quoted at 10%, but with either bilateral V1 or concurrent V1, V2, or V3 this may increase to 25% or even higher. Patients with V2 or V3 PWS without any involvement of the V1 skin, however, are not at risk for SWS. Care needs to be taken to allow for individual anatomic variations in the distribution of V1 and V2 at the internal or external canthus of the eye, so called "watershed areas," as it may be difficult to ascertain for sure the exact cutoff between V zones (Figure 8-2).

Early ophthalmologic evaluation is appropriate in infants with facial PWS involving the V1 or "watershed" distribution. Neuroimaging consisting of magnetic resonance imaging (MRI) with gadolinium enhancement may be helpful in assessing neurologic involvement. However, a negative study during the neonatal period does not exclude SWS with certainty, as changes can continue to evolve, particularly during the first 2 years of life.

Early subtle changes on MRI can include an enlarged choroid plexus or a pattern of local accelerated myelination. Typical neuroimaging changes include visualization of the pial vascular malformation; cerebral atrophy; and calcifications of the leptomeninges, the abnormal cortex, and the underlying white matter. Affected patients usually manifest clinically with seizures before 2 years of age. Other manifestations include brain hypoxia, neuronal loss, disturbed regional cerebral blood flow, and a risk of contralateral hemiplegia. Developmental delay of cognitive skills may occur to varying degrees. Migraine headaches are common. Acute or chronic glaucoma remains a constant concern and requires ongoing ophthalmologic follow-up. Prophylactic antiseizure medications are advocated by some specialists for at-risk infants, though this practice is controversial and not standard of care. Management is focused on close follow-up for vision, motor, and psychomotor development and reduction of facial disfigurement throughout life.

PWS on extremities may be associated with venous varicosities and soft tissue and bone hyperplasia, with or without lymphatic malformations, termed Klippel-Trenaunay syndrome. If AVMs are concurrent, the term *Parkes Weber syndrome* is used. Extremity PWS should be followed carefully for limb-length inequality, localized thrombosis, pain, and functional impact. Significant lesions may require multispecialty management including dermatology, orthopedics, laser surgery, interventional radiology, plastic surgery, and interdisciplinary vascular lesion clinics.

Suggested Readings

Enjolras O, Garzon MC. Vascular stains, malformations, and tumors. *Neonatal Dermatology.* 2nd ed. Philadelphia, PA: Saunders Elsevier; 2008:343-368.

Enjolras O, Riche MC, Merland JJ. Facial port-wine stains and Sturge-Weber syndrome. *Pediatrics.* 1985;76(1):48-51.

Tallman B, Tan OT, Morelli JG, et al. Location of port-wine stains and the likelihood of ophthalmic and/or central nervous system complications. *Pediatrics.* 1991;87(3):323-327.

SECTION II

NEVI AND PHOTOPROTECTION

WHAT SUNSCREEN SHOULD I RECOMMEND TO MY PATIENTS AND HOW CAN I BALANCE SUN PROTECTION WITH ENSURING THAT THEY RECEIVE ENOUGH VITAMIN D?

Lisa Arkin, MD

Background

Skin cancer may be the most preventable malignancy as its association with exposure to ultraviolet (UV) radiation is well established. The sun emits a spectrum of UV radiation that is arbitrarily subdivided into UV-A (wavelengths 400 to 315 nm), UV-B (wavelengths 315 to 290 nm), and UV-C (wavelengths 290 to 200 nm). UV-A and UV-B are known to directly damage DNA by producing aberrant, unstable covalent bonds and generating highly reactive chemical intermediates that predispose to carcinogenesis. In addition, all wavelengths of UV radiation accelerate the aging process by directly damaging collagen in the skin.

Sunscreen was developed to protect against these harmful effects. The sun protection factor of sunscreen, or SPF, is defined as the amount of UV radiation required to produce sunburn on skin *with sunscreen* compared to skin *without sunscreen*. This means that a woman wearing SPF 30 sunscreen would take 30 times longer to burn than she would without any sunscreen.

Sunscreen: What Are the Choices?

There are two types of sunscreens, those that scatter UV radiation (physical blockers) and those that absorb it (chemical absorbers). Physical blockers, which are also called sun blocks, are composed of opaque particles of inorganic material that scatter UV light before it can penetrate the skin. These sunscreens typically contain zinc oxide or titanium dioxide; they protect against both UV-A and UV-B radiation (the wavelengths associated with carcinogenesis). While the original formulations of physical blockers remained white when applied to skin, they are now compounded into ultrafine nanoparticles that blend into the skin but retain their UV-blocking effects. In contrast, chemical absorbers, which are also referred to as sunscreens, are organic particles that absorb UV-A and UV-B, converting them into harmless intermediates before they can damage skin. They typically contain multiple ingredients such as benzophenone, cinnamates, or salicylates.

The most recent policy statement on ultraviolet radiation from the American Academy of Pediatrics recommends sun avoidance and sun protective clothing for all children and adolescents. In children older than 6 months, the use of sunscreen with SPF more than 15 is recommended. Both physical blockers and chemical absorbers are effective, but only when applied every 2 hours or immediately after exposure to water. The recommended dose of sunscreen is 2 mg/cm^2, which amounts to approximately 1 oz per sitting for a school-aged child. For infants younger than 6 months, sun avoidance and protective clothing should be first line, with use of sunscreen as necessary to sun exposed areas including the face and hands.

Sunscreen Has Known Benefits…
But Are There Risks?

Among its known benefits, sunscreen has been shown to protect against the harmful effects of UV radiation, photoaging, and the development of squamous cell carcinoma (Table 9-1). To date, there are no studies that have proven that sunscreen prevents basal cell carcinomas or melanoma, even though numerous studies *have* documented the relationship between intense intermittent sun exposure (including childhood sunburns) and the development of these malignancies. The reason for this is unclear. Some have argued that the predisposition to these particular skin cancers involves not only sun exposure but also a host of other unknown factors that were not accounted for in the trials. In children, we do know that an increased number of melanocytic nevi correlates with both sun exposure *and* an increased risk for melanoma.

In addition, in recent years, several in vitro and animal studies have raised the question of whether sunscreen may in fact be potentially harmful. These concerns center on whether sunscreens have adverse hormonal effects or may be potentially mutagenic. First, some have suggested that the compounds used in chemical sunscreens—among them benzophenone, octyl-methoxycinnamate, and 3,4 methyl-benzylidene—have estrogenic properties that might disrupt hormone levels. However, the only study performed in humans demonstrated that daily sunscreen application did not alter the levels of endogenous reproductive hormones in men and women. Others have suggested that both physical and chemical sunscreens may amplify free radicals, resulting in DNA damage and increasing the risk for cancer. To date, these studies have not been performed on human skin and there is no convincing evidence that they are clinically relevant. In the general population, sunscreen has been used for decades without adverse effects and has an excellent safety profile.

Table 9-1
Known Benefits of Sunscreen

- Protects from UV radiation
- Prevents squamous cell carcinoma
- Prevents signs of aging
- Sunscreen has not been shown to prevent the development of melanoma or basal cell carcinoma

What About the Vitamin D Question?

In addition, there are some who believe that sunscreen may be harmful because it reduces vitamin D production. The vast majority of de-novo vitamin D synthesis occurs in the skin through the action of UV-B radiation, which converts cholesterol precursors into vitamin D_3. In the absence of oral supplementation, strict sun protection will produce a state of vitamin D deficiency. In children, the most well-known complication of this is rickets, but emerging evidence has also suggested that vitamin D may play a role in maintaining innate immunity and preventing the development of autoimmune diseases, including multiple sclerosis, systemic lupus erythematosus, rheumatoid arthritis, and diabetes mellitus; infectious and cardiovascular diseases; and some forms of cancer.

Should This Impact Our Recommendations to Patients Regarding Sun Protection?

The answer to this question is relatively straightforward. A multitude of factors affect the amount of UV-B radiation available for vitamin D synthesis, including skin pigmentation, body mass, cloud cover, air pollution, season, degree of skin coverage, and UV protection in the form of sunscreen. Melanin, an insoluble substance that gives skin and hair its pigment, is the body's own natural defense against UV radiation. It absorbs UV radiation and dissipates the energy as heat. As a result, those with darker skin require 5 to 10 times more exposure to generate similar amounts of vitamin D relative to those with lighter skin. Geographical location is also an important consideration. A recent study found that people who lived in Boston, MA, could not synthesize sufficient vitamin D in the winter regardless of how long they were outside. For all of these reasons, the American Academy of Pediatrics recommends oral supplementation of vitamin D and continued sun protection. All infants and children, including adolescents, should have a minimum daily intake of 400 IU of vitamin D beginning soon after birth. Many foods are fortified with vitamin D (Table 9-2) and oral vitamin D supplements are readily available over the counter. Children at risk for hypovitaminosis D due to low intake or underlying systemic disease require appropriate laboratory evaluation including 25(OH)D levels.

Table 9-2

Vitamin D Content of Foods

Food	Vitamin D Content (IU)
Cow's milk	3 to 40/L
Fortified milk/infant formula	400/L
Fortified orange juice/soy milk/rice milk	400/L
Margarine, fortified	429/100 g
Butter	35/100 g
Shrimp	152/100 g
Cooked salmon/mackerel	345 to 360/100 g
Yogurt	89/100 g

IU indicates international unit

Data adapted from http://www.nal.usda.gov/fnic/foodcomp/Data/Other/vit_d99.pdf

Summary

The safest way to protect our pediatric patients is to recommend both strict sun protection and daily oral vitamin D supplementation. Sun-protective clothing including shirts, pants, wide brimmed hats, and UV protective sunglasses are safe, relatively inexpensive, and available through a variety of outlets (www.coolibar.com, www.solartex.com). Sun avoidance strategies and protective clothing should be first line whenever possible for all babies less than 6 months. For all other children and adolescents, a combination of sun-protective clothing and sunscreen with an SPF more than 15 is recommended, with reapplication every 2 hours or immediately after water exposure. Children should also stay in the shade whenever possible. Skin cancer prevention is a lifelong effort that must begin in childhood.

Suggested Readings

Balk SJ; Council on Environmental Health, Section on Dermatology. Ultraviolet radiation: a hazard to children and adolescents. *Pediatrics*. 2011;127(3):e791-e817.

Delco VA. Sunscreens. In: Bolognia JL, et al (eds). *Dermatology*. Spain: Mosby Elsevier; 2008:2035-2041.

Janjua NR, Mogensen B, Andersson AM, et al. Systemic absorption of the sunscreens benzophenone-3, octyl-methoxycinnamate, and 3-(4-methyl-benzylidene) camphor after whole-body topical application and reproductive hormone levels in humans. *J Invest Dermatol*. 2004;123(1):57-61.

Misra M, Pacaud D, Petryk A, et al. Vitamin D deficiency in children and its management: review of current knowledge and recommendations. *Pediatrics*. 2008;122(2):398-417.

Reichrath J. Skin cancer prevention and UV-protection: how to avoid vitamin D-deficiency? *Br J Dermatol*. 2009;161(Suppl 3):54-60.

Wagner CL, Greer FR; American Academy of Pediatrics Section on Breastfeeding; American Academy of Pediatrics Committee on Nutrition. Prevention of rickets and vitamin D deficiency in infants, children and adolescents. *Pediatrics*. 2008;122(5):1142-1152.

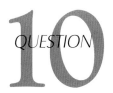

WHAT DO I NEED TO KNOW ABOUT ACQUIRED NEVI?

Kara N. Shah, MD, PhD

Acquired melanocytic nevi (moles) are very common in children. They represent benign proliferations of melanocytes, the pigment-producing cells in the skin. They usually are noted to develop after 1 to 2 years of age; melanocytic nevi that develop within the first year of life are generally best regarded as congenital nevi. The number of acquired nevi increases with age through adolescence and early adulthood; therefore, it is *normal* for children and adolescents to develop new moles.

Risk factors for the development of acquired nevi include fair skin type with blue or green eyes; blonde or red hair; inability to tan; sun exposure, in particular intermittent, high-intensity sun exposure; freckling; and prior sunburn or cutaneous blistering disease. Immunosuppression secondary to chemotherapy or stem cell, bone marrow, or solid organ transplantation is also associated with the development of acquired nevi. In addition, in some families there appears to be a genetic tendency to develop large number of melanocytic nevi. Children with Turner syndrome or Noonan syndrome also tend to develop high nevus counts.

Most acquired melanocytic nevi are small (<6 mm in diameter), symmetric, and evenly pigmented (Figure 10-1). They may be flat (junctional nevi) or raised (compound and dermal nevi). Acquired melanocytic nevi on the scalp may have an "eclipse" appearance with a lighter, raised central component and a more darkly pigmented peripheral component (Figure 10-2). Melanocytic nevi on the scalp may manifest some histological atypia when biopsied and appear to be associated with the development of dysplastic nevi elsewhere on the body. In general, I do not excise "eclipse" scalp nevi unless they develop concerning clinical features.

Acquired nevi may be confused with freckles (ephelides), which are non-nevoid melanocytic lesions that typically are small (<1 to 2 mm in diameter), lightly pigmented, poorly circumscribed macules located on chronically sun-exposed areas such as the face. Unlike melanocytic nevi, freckles accentuate with sun exposure and fade during the winter. Acquired melanocytic nevi may also be confused with small café-au-lait macules or with

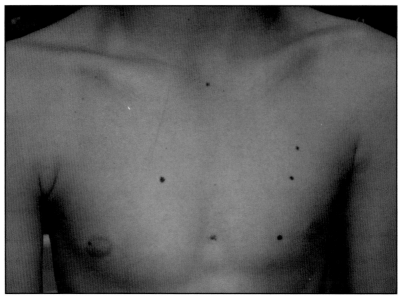

Figure 10-1. Typical acquired melanocytic nevi in an adolescent.

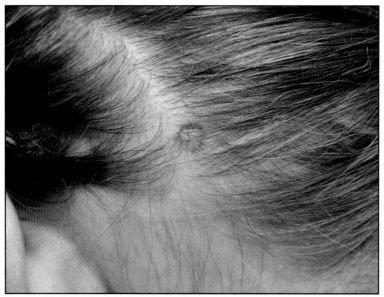

Figure 10-2. Typical "eclipse" acquired melanocytic nevus on the scalp.

lentigines, which are small, darkly and homogeneously pigmented, well-demarcated non-nevoid melanocytic macules that may occur singly or in large numbers on the skin and mucous membranes. Lentigines are not related to sun exposure. Isolated lentigines in children (lentigo simplex) are of no clinical significance. The presence of numerous lentigines should raise the suspicion of an associated syndrome such as LEOPARD (lentigines [multiple], electrocardiographic abnormalities, ocular hypertelorism, pulmonary stenosis, abnormalities of genitalia, retardation of growth, and deafness [sensorineural]) syndrome, Carney complex, or Peutz-Jeghers syndrome.

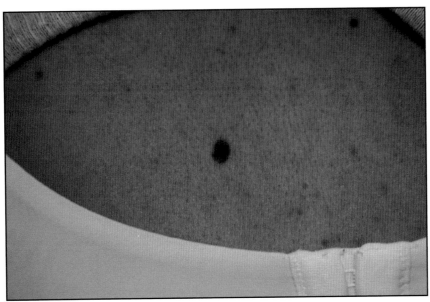

Figure 10-3. Dysplastic nevus.

Although more common in adults, some children may develop dysplastic nevi, which are acquired melanocytic nevi with atypical clinical and/or histologic features. Clinically, dysplastic nevi often have a "fried egg" appearance, with a raised, more darkly pigmented central component and a more lightly pigmented, irregular, ill-defined border (Figure 10-3). They are usually more than 6 mm in diameter and have irregular pigmentation with shades of brown and pink. They most commonly appear on the torso. Histologically, dysplastic nevi manifest cytological and architectural atypia. The presence of numerous dysplastic nevi confers an increased risk for the development of melanoma, although not typically within a pre-existing dysplastic nevus. Although controversial, it does not appear that the majority of dysplastic nevi are premalignant or evolve into melanoma.

The vast majority of acquired nevi in children are benign. The development of progressive changes in the appearance of a melanocytic nevus raises the concern for the development of a dysplastic nevus or, very rarely, melanoma. The ABCDE mnemonic is helpful in the clinical evaluation of moles in children: asymmetry; (irregular) borders; color variegation (two or more colors, including black, white, red, blue, and brown or shades of brown); diameter (>6 mm or the size of a pencil eraser); and evolution, enlargement, or elevation of any part of the mole. The development of one or more of these changes in a melanocytic nevus indicates that the melanocytic nevus warrants re-evaluation; although it does not indicate that the melanocytic nevus is dysplastic or premalignant. The development of bleeding, pain, pruritus, or ulceration associated with an acquired melanocytic nevus also warrants further evaluation. In addition, evaluation of any melanocytic nevus that clinically appears very different from the majority of the other nevi present (the "ugly duckling" mole) is also recommended. Referral to a dermatologist is recommended for further evaluation of any acquired nevus that has developed a sudden increase in size; asymmetry or irregular changes in pigmentation; or inflammation, bleeding, or ulceration. In many cases, only close clinical follow-up with photodocumentation is appropriate; in other cases, biopsy or excision of the nevus for histological evaluation may be recommended. I find the use of photodocumentation in the clinical follow-up of melanocytic nevi to be extremely valuable as it allows for both caregivers and clinical providers to better monitor selected melanocytic nevi for the development of a significant change in the appearance of any nevus that is being clinically observed.

Biopsy or excision of an atypical melanocytic nevus allows for evaluation of the histological features of the melanocytic nevus and can differentiate between benign melanocytic nevi (junctional, compound, and dermal), dysplastic nevi (often graded as mild, moderate, or severe), and malignant melanoma. In general, I do not recommend additional treatment of dysplastic nevi with only mild atypia; those with moderate or severe atypia I usually re-excise to ensure complete removal and prevent recurrence if only part of the nevus was initially biopsied. In rare circumstances, the histological interpretation of a melanocytic nevus may be exceedingly difficult with features of significant atypia but without a clear diagnosis of malignant melanoma; in these cases, the melanocytic nevus may be descriptively characterized as a "melanocytic tumor of uncertain malignant potential" or other similar terminology. As the descriptor implies, these unusual melanocytic nevi have an unpredictable natural history and are best managed by a dermatologist with expertise in pigmented lesions.

Several distinct clinical variants of benign acquired melanocytic nevi may be seen in children, including halo nevi, Spitz nevi, and blue nevi.

Halo nevi are relatively common in children and represent the development of a benign host lymphocytic inflammatory response to an existing melanocytic nevus. Immune-mediated destruction of melanocytes results in a peripheral zone of depigmentation around the melanocytic nevus and often to eventual disappearance of the entire nevus (Figure 10-4). Halo nevi are often seen in association with vitiligo, and the pathophysiology of these two phenomena is likely related. Halo nevi have also been reported in association with Turner syndrome. Unless the clinical appearance of the melanocytic nevus itself is atypical or worrisome, halo nevi in children do not need to be biopsied or excised, and there is no association with an increased risk for the development of melanoma.

The Spitz nevus typically appears as a pink papule located on the head or neck (Figure 10-5). Spitz nevi may initially grow very rapidly, but most remain less than 1 cm in greatest diameter. Some Spitz nevi are pigmented and manifest as a darkly pigmented macule or papule that may clinically resemble a simple acquired melanocytic nevus. On clinical examination of a Spitz nevus with dermoscopy, or handheld epiluminescence microscopy, a characteristic starburst pattern of the pigment network may be appreciated. Spitz nevi typically have a characteristic histology, but occasionally may mimic melanoma. Although controversial, I typically recommend complete excision of all Spitz nevi to prevent future confusion with an evolving melanoma. Spitz nevi that exhibit atypical histologic features may be referred to as an "atypical Spitz tumor" or "Spitz tumor with atypia"; although these likely represent a benign variant of the Spitz nevus, referral to a dermatologist with expertise in pigmented lesions for further evaluation and management, including complete surgical excision, is advised.

The blue nevus usually presents as a small, blue-gray macule or papule and most commonly is located on the head, buttocks, or distal extremities. The histology of a common blue nevus characteristically manifests a dermal proliferation of spindled melanoctyes. Malignant degeneration within a blue nevus is rare, and most do not need to be excised unless worrisome clinical features are present.

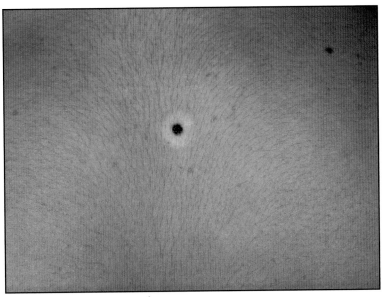

Figure 10-4. Halo nevus phenomenon.

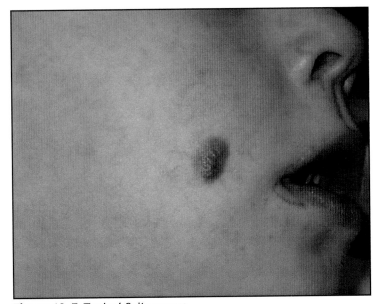

Figure 10-5. Typical Spitz nevus.

Melanoma fortunately is very rare in children, although the incidence is increasing, in particular during adolescence. The majority of melanomas in children (>70%) are estimated to arise de novo and not from a pre-existing nevus. Risk factors for the development of melanoma are similar to those for acquired melanocytic nevi, and in particular include a history of prolonged immunosuppression, chemotherapy, or radiation therapy. Risk factors also include the presence of dysplastic nevi, a high count (>100) of common acquired nevi, melanoma in a first-degree relative, and previous diagnosis of melanoma.

A genetic, familial predisposition to the development of melanoma may be seen in the familial atypical mole melanoma syndrome (FAMMS), which is associated with mutations in the genes CDKN2A, CDK4, and CMM1. FAMMS accounts for approximately 10% of melanomas in adults but a very low percentage of melanoma seen in children.

All children and adolescents and their caregivers should receive education on the importance of sun protection and avoidance of excess sun exposure, including avoidance of tanning beds. General recommendations include limiting the amount of sun exposure during the hours or 10 am and 2 pm, use of sun-protective clothing (including hats and sunglasses), and appropriate use of a broad-spectrum sunscreen. Several companies now market sun-protective clothing, including swimwear and shirts, that offer a universal protection factor of 50 (equivalent to an SPF of 50). Frequent application every 2 hours of a broad-spectrum sunscreen during periods of sun exposure and in particular after swimming or excessive sweating is recommended. In general, I recommend a sunscreen containing zinc oxide and titanium dioxide, which provide broad-spectrum protection and are suitable for use in all children, including those with sensitive skin.

Suggested Readings

Gallagher RP, McLean DI. The epidemiology of acquired melanocytic nevi. A brief review. *Dermatol Clin.* 1995; 13(3):595-603.

Gallagher RP, Rivers JK, Lee TK, Bajdik CD, McLean DI, Coldman AJ. Broad-spectrum sunscreen use and the development of new nevi in white children: a randomized controlled trial. *JAMA.* 2000;283(22):2955-2960.

Schaffer JV. Pigmented lesions in children: when to worry. *Curr Opin Pediatr.* 2007;19(4):430-440.

Whiteman DC, Brown RM, Purdie DM, Hughes MC. Melanocytic nevi in very young children: the role of phenotype, sun exposure, and sun protection. *J Am Acad Dermatol.* 2005;52(1):40-47.

HOW SHOULD I MANAGE LARGE NEVI?

Leslie Castelo-Soccio, MD, PhD

Large nevi include 2 groups of melanocytic nevi: large congenital melanocytic nevi and acquired nevi over 6 mm.

Large congenital nevi are nevi defined as those larger than 20 cm in size (10 cm in the scalp; Figure 11-1). These lesions should be referred to a dermatologist because they can be difficult to follow and they often develop confusing verrucous papules and variegated color within the lesion. They can be particularly challenging to follow when they arise with multiple colors rather than a uniform color. Risk for malignant transformation is about 2.5% over a lifetime with most melanomas (approximately 70%) occurring before the age of 10. Nevi greater than 40 cm in size have the highest risk for developing melanoma. Clinically they should be followed closely with serial photographs, dermatoscopy, and clinical examinations. Clinical examinations should include palpation since many melanomas develop deep within the dermis and cannot be visualized. Management also includes evaluation for neurocutaneous melanosis (NCM) and decision about surgical intervention.

NCM is defined as melanocytes within the central nervous system (CNS) and occurs in about 10% of patients with giant congenital nevi. It is more common in patients with large congenital nevi, but also occurs in patients with smaller nevi in midline posterior axial region with multiple satellite lesions (usually greater than 20) or with more than three congenital nevi. Symptoms of NCM typically arise from the obstructive or compressive effects of the melanocytes in these regions. Evaluation for headaches, seizures, hydrocephalus, vomiting, developmental delay, and cranial nerve palsies is critical to monitoring patients with large congenital nevi. Structural anomalies such as Dandy-Walker malformations have also been reported.

Because the majority of patients with NCM are asymptomatic, there is debate about the utility of magnetic resonance imaging (MRI). If patients are asymptomatic, does identifying the NCM alter management? Many say no and so only suggest screening if the patient is symptomatic. MRI may also be beneficial if a large excision is to be undertaken. I often caution patients and families that if they have NCM, then putting them through serial excision may not significantly reduce their overall risk of

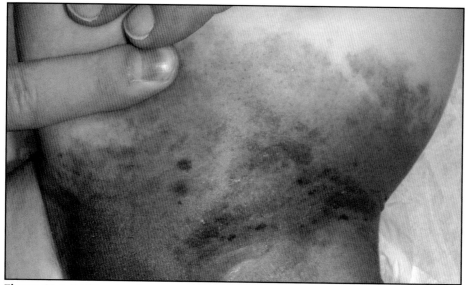

Figure 11-1. Bathing trunk nevus with multiple areas of hyperpigmentation.

melanoma because the melanocytes within the CNS that cannot be resected could also undergo malignant degeneration. MRI of the complete brain and spine is the study of choice. The most frequent MRI finding is the presence of increased signal on T1. These areas of increased signal represent accumulation of melanocytic cells. The most frequent areas of infiltration are the anterior temporal area, the cerebellum, and close to the amygdala. Malignant transformation is suggested by the presence of necrosis, hemorrhage, edema, or growth. The cerebrospinal fluid of neonates with NCM may reveal protein, decreased sugar, and a normal cell count, although melanin-filled cells are sometimes found in the cerebrospinal fluid. If NCM is identified, the patient should be referred to a neurologist familiar with managing these patients. Once symptomatic, patients with NCM have a poor prognosis. In a series of 71 cases, mortality occurred in 77% of patients with a median survival of 6.5 months after symptoms occurred and median age of death of 4.5 years.

Surgery for large congenital nevi is also controversial. While removing lesions reduces the risk of melanoma, the risk may not decrease it to zero because melanocytes can track deep and can be present in the CNS. Surgery brings with it the risk of sedation, risk of long-term scarring, and the possibility that if the entire lesion is not removed that the surgical scar can obscure change and make clinical follow-up challenging. Many argue that with thorough examinations and a low threshold for biopsy of a new nodule or darker segment within the nevus, surgery is not necessary. Since congenital nevi can be located on any part of the body, surgery is also dependent on body site. Many areas are inoperable or would require extensive skin grafting or skin expanders. Many patients in consultation with their surgeons will opt for partial removals. Even after removal, the management is to carefully follow the scar for changes in color or size, changes in texture, formation of nodules, and development of symptoms such as itching or bleeding. Full skin examinations should also be completed. Lifelong follow-up is essential especially in patients who have had an excision.

The second group of large nevi is acquired melanocytic nevi. Clinically, dysplastic nevi are larger than 6 mm in size, are irregularly bordered, and have irregular pigmentation. The lifetime risk of melanoma in these lesions has been reported to be as high as 10%. Clinicians need to assess the characteristics of the large acquired nevus in question to decide on management and to assess if the nevus is clinically atypical. One of the simplest first steps is to look at the lesion in the context of the child's other moles. If the nevus in question looks like the other moles or is a "signature mole," it can usually be followed over time for changes in color, size, symmetry, and symptoms (itch, bleeding). The exceptions to this is if the lesion is occurring in a child with a significant family history of melanoma or dysplastic nevi; if the child has greater than 50 melanocytic nevi, some of which are clinically atypical; or if the nevus is located in a special site such as the scalp, genital area, or acral regions. There is a lower threshold for biopsy in these patients. Blue nevi, lentigos, Spitz nevi, and dermatofibromas should be considered in the differential of large clinically atypical moles. Management requires thorough examination and photography, patient education, regular follow-up, and sometimes excisional biopsy of representative suspicious lesions particularly if they are on the scalp or acral areas. It is frequently helpful for the clinician to re-evaluate in a few months from first detection to see that the mole is stable. Daily evaluations by the patient or family are not necessary since it is difficult to assess for change over time by doing this and can make families anxious. But the moles should be followed monthly. It is important to remember that many patients simply have an increased number of banal-appearing moles in the absence of atypical nevi. Photos can be helpful to objectively look for change on a monthly basis. If the lesion is an "ugly duckling" (does not look like the patient's other moles), assess what makes it look different.

Simple questions to ask yourself when you are evaluating moles include the following: Does the lesion have multiple colors? Is the lesion raised in some areas but flat in others? Does the lesion have an odd, asymmetric shape? Is the lesion greater than 6 mm? Is the lesion bleeding or itchy? If the answer is yes to any of these questions, this is likely a clinically dysplastic nevi or possibly a melanoma and biopsy should be highly considered. Dermoscopy can be used to evaluate, however, the clinical use of this method relies on the expertise of the individual. In trained individuals, dermoscopy can improve accuracy in identifying atypical nevi from banal nevi. A recent change should alert the clinician to consider an excision or biopsy to rule out the development of malignant melanoma. All patients diagnosed with one or more atypical nevi should undergo a complete cutaneous examination, which includes the scalp and mucous membranes. Several studies show that regular cutaneous examinations combined with photography decrease the number of biopsies and lead to earlier diagnosis of melanoma. Patients should be taught self-examination to detect changes. Patients should be educated about avoiding UV-emitting tanning, excessive sun exposure, and the proper use of sunscreens and protective clothing (see Question 10).

Suggested Readings

Grobb JJ, Bonerandi JJ. The "ugly duckling" sign: identification of the common characteristics of nevi in an individual as a basis for melanoma screening. *Arch Dermatol*. 1998;134(1):103-104.

Marks R. Epidemiology of melanoma. *Clin Exp Derm*. 2000;25:459-468.

Price HN, Schaffer JV. Congenital melanocytic nevi when to worry and how to treat: facts and controversies. *Clin Dermatol.* 2010;28(3):293-302.

Scope A, Dusza SW, Halpern AC, Rabinovitz H, Braun RP, Zalaudek I. The "ugly duckling" sign: agreement between observers. *Arch Dermatol.* 2008;144(1):58-64.

Slutsky JB, Barr JM, Femia AN, Marghoob AA. Large congenital melanocytic nevi: associated risks and management considerations. *Semin Cutan Med Surg.* 2010;29(2):79-84.

Suh KY, Bolongnia JL. Signature nevi. *J Am Acad Dermatol.* 2009;60(3):508-514.

SHOULD MOLES ON THE HANDS, FEET, AND SCALP ALWAYS BE REMOVED?

Patrick McMahon, MD

Although moles (nevi) on the hands, feet, and scalp were routinely removed in the past, this practice is no longer recommended. In this review, I will outline the reasons in support of clinical monitoring for the majority of these moles as well as stress certain clinical scenarios where referral and possibly a diagnostic biopsy or removal would be warranted.

Previously, moles on the palms, soles, and scalp were thought to have an increased risk of becoming malignant. This may have been because these moles, now considered "nevi of special sites" do have some features that microscopically can resemble melanoma.

Although the incidence of melanoma is reportedly increasing, the annual transformation of a single mole into a melanoma is as low as 0.0005% in patients under 40 years old.[1] Lending further credence to the argument against routine excision of these moles is the case of a recurrent nevus. If a mole is excised, recurrence of pigment within the scar presents a challenging clinical scenario, even if the original mole was deemed benign. These recurrent nevi are difficult to monitor clinically since the pigment may be irregularly distributed within a scar and upon repeat biopsy they have an altered architecture. For this reason, recurrent nevi have been called *pseudomelanoma*; a murky predicament that can be encountered less by a more measured approach. In sum, as stated in the Hurwitz textbook of clinical pediatric dermatology, "prophylactic excision of all nevi in these locations is unwarranted."[1(p207)]

There exist clinical situations wherein referral, and possibly a biopsy, of moles on the hands, feet, and scalp is warranted. As with moles on any part of the body, clinical features of **a**symmetry, irregular **b**orders, changing **c**olor, **d**iameter greater than 6 mm, and **e**nlargement (or **e**volution) should be screened for at each visit. These features, which can be suggestive of a malignant melanoma, have been called the ABCDE signs. If these signs, or others such as bleeding, itching, ulceration, or pain, are present, a prompt referral to a dermatologist is warranted. Other risk factors that I routinely consider when making the decision whether or not to perform a biopsy include a family, and certainly personal,

Figure 12-1. Irregularly pigmented nevus with dark pigment on the dorsal hand, which on removal was found to be an atypical spindle cell nevus.

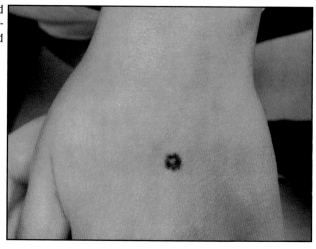

history of melanoma. It should be noted that as children grow, their benign moles will grow along with them; therefore, in the pediatric setting, absolute change in size alone should not dictate the need for a biopsy.

Moles on the Hands and Feet (Acral Nevi)

When evaluating moles on the hands and feet, there are 2 settings in which I monitor a patient more closely and have a lower threshold to biopsy. These include (1) acral nevi in a darkly pigmented patient and (2) pigmented nail bands especially in a lightly pigmented patient. The first situation is because, although rare, malignant melanoma in darkly pigmented individuals is found most commonly in areas with less pigment (ie, the mucous membranes, palms, soles, and nail beds). Therefore, all moles on the palms, soles, and nail beds in this population require close monitoring. Any atypical or changing lesion would deserve a biopsy (Figure 12-1). The second setting in which a mole on the hands and feet grabs my attention is the case of a pigmented nail streak (melanonychia striata). Although a benign melanocytic proliferation within the nail matrix can produce a pigmented nail band, there are certain clues found on physical examination that would be cause for concern. These signs include a particularly dark, broad, and expanding streak or extension of pigment onto the proximal or lateral nail folds (the latter being the so-called Hutchinson sign). Since the nail plate grows out over time, expansion of a pigmented band may be noted by comparing the diameter of the distal portion to the diameter proximally. If the width is larger proximally, this indicates that the underlying melanocytic lesion is enlarging. Overall, benign pigmentation of the nails is less common in white individuals, so any nail pigment noted in this population deserves close attention.

A Note on Congenital Melanocytic Nevi

Congenital melanocytic nevi (CMN) present a unique case, especially in cosmetically sensitive locations such as the scalp, hairline, or dorsal hands. These nevi tend to be dark, thicker, and contain coarse overlying hairs, which can be troubling to the patient

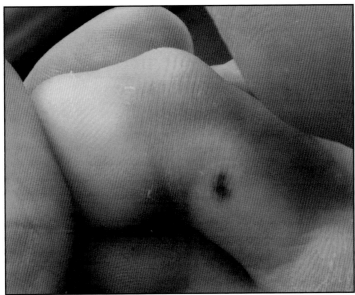

Figure 12-2. Normal benign nevus on the toe with regular pigment following the skin markings.

(see Question 13 for a full discussion). Although small (<1.5 cm in diameter) and medium CMNs (1.5 to 20 cm) have been found to hold a very low risk of malignant transformation, they can be disfiguring or embarrassing for some patients.[2] For this reason, I have referred adolescent patients to plastic surgeons to discuss treatment options that may include a staged excision, depending on the size.

Summary

Routine excision of moles on the hands, feet, and scalp is not recommended (Figure 12-2). As with all pigmented lesions, careful clinical monitoring for worrisome changes is of utmost importance. Certain unique clinical settings, detailed previously, include acral nevi, pigmented nail bands (melanonychia striata), and CMN.

References

1. Paller AS, Mancini AJ. *Hurwitz Clinical Pediatric Dermatology: A Textbook of Skin Disorders of Childhood and Adolescence*, 3rd ed. Philadelphia, PA: Elsevier Saunders; 2006.
2. Slutsky JB, Barr JM, Femia AN, Marghoob AA. Large congenital melanocytic nevi: associated risks and management considerations. *Semin Cutan Med Surg.* 2010;29(2):79-84.

13

DO ALL CONGENITAL NEVI NEED TO BE REFERRED TO A DERMATOLOGIST?

Leslie Castelo-Soccio, MD, PhD

The short answer is no. Not all congenital nevi need to be referred to a dermatologist. Two percent to 4% of all children have pigmented lesions at birth. Congenital nevi occur in all ethnicities and malignant transformation can occur regardless of background skin pigmentation. Congenital nevi are typically present at birth or within a few months of birth. They can become visible up to 2 years of age. Congenital nevi are commonly classified based on size, which can be helpful in determining referral. Size is based on the largest diameter of the nevus in adulthood. Because nevi enlarge in proportion to the child's growth, the final diameter can be predicted by estimating a size increase from infancy to adulthood by a factor of about 2 on the head and factor of 3 on the body. The greatest concerns for transformation are giant congenital nevi and these are typically nevi that should be referred. Giant or large congenital nevi are larger than 20 cm in size (see Figure 11-1). The exception is nevi on the scalp, which are considered large if greater than 10 cm in size.

Large congenital nevi are rare and difficult to follow. All large congenital nevi should be referred to a dermatologist since over time they may develop variegated color and can develop verrucous papules within the lesion itself, which make following clinically for changes in size, shape, or color challenging. Melanoma often presents with a new papular, nodular, or ulcerated area within a giant congenital nevus. Any distinct, localized change in color or texture should be evaluated immediately. Dermatologists will follow serially with photographs and clinically examination visually and with palpation and have a low threshold to biopsy. The risk of malignant transformation in these lesions is high and melanomas can occur in childhood. Seventy percent of melanomas that occur within large congenital nevi occur before the age of 10. The risk of transformation is approximately 2.5% to 5%, although some authors quote as high as 11%. Typically these higher percentages refer to nevi that are greater than 40 cm in diameter.

Congenital nevi larger than 40 cm with multiple satellite lesions and location on the posterior axis have the highest risk of malignant transformation. Having 20 or more

Figure 13-1. Congenital mole on the dorsal hand that would be very difficult to remove entirely.

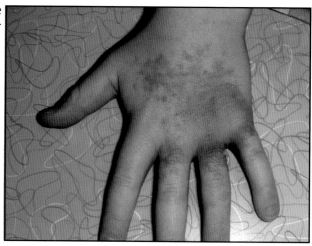

satellite nevi, whether or not associated with a giant axial congenital nevus, is actually the most predictive of NCM. Patients with NCM have abnormal melanocytes clustered in the brain and spinal cord.

NCM can be detected by magnetic resonance imaging (MRI). NCM may not be symptomatic and there is debate about screening MRIs if patients are asymptomatic. If screening MRI is to be performed, it may be best to test between birth and 4 months of age before mylenization occurs since myelin can obscure more subtle deposits of melanocytes. However, because neurologic manifestations typically occur before the age of 2, some argue against screening unless symptomatic. Others suggest waiting until 6 months of age when the sedation risk of an MRI is diminished. Typical manifestations of NCM are related to the space-occupying effects of melanocytes in the brain or spinal cord and can include headaches, seizures, hydrocephalus, vomiting, and developmental delay. Structural anomalies such as Dandy-Walker malformations have also been reported in patients with symptomatic NCM. The most frequent MRI finding is the presence of increased signal on T1. These areas of increased signal represent accumulation of melanocytic cells. The most frequent areas of infiltration are the anterior temporal area, the cerebellum, and close to the amygdala. MRI may reveal the presence of an arachnoid cyst in the spinal cord. Malignant transformation is suggested by the presence of necrosis, hemorrhage, edema, and growth. Contrast enhancement by computed tomography can be helpful if there is concern about malignant transformation. Patients who develop symptomatic NCM have a poor survival rate. Small case studies show that the majority of patients survive only 6.5 months after initial symptoms begin. Neurology and neuro-oncology should be consulted if MRI suggests NCM in a patient with symptoms.

Management of giant congenital nevi is complex. Surgical excision does decrease the incidence of melanoma. However, in most instances, excision is only partial and even total resection does not eliminate the risk of melanoma because melanocytes can be deep or present in other sites like the central nervous system. Also many are inoperable (Figure 13-1). Surgery comes with significant risks of scarring. Many argue that given the low incidence of melanoma overall that clinically following patients with serial examinations and photographs is superior to surgery. Treatment decisions must take into account the size and location of the nevus, presence or absence of NCM, symptoms or changes as well as patient and family preferences.

Small and intermediate congenital nevi are defined as those less than 1.5 cm (small) and greater than 1.5 cm but less than 20 cm (intermediate). The risk of malignant transformation in small or intermediate lesions is probably less than 1% over a lifetime with the majority occurring in teenagers. Over a period of 30 years at Massachusetts General Hospital and New York University Pigmented Lesion Clinics, no patient younger than 20 years was found to have a melanoma within a congenital nevus smaller than 5 cm in diameter. Small and intermediate congenital nevi do not need to be referred unless they are significantly variegated in color; located in special sites such as the nails, hands or feet, or genital region; there is a significant family history of melanoma; or they have undergone significant change over time. It is important to note that congenital nevi grow with the child and that over time they frequently become elevated, textured, and darker. They also can develop coarse hair. Congenital nevi can range from tan to black in color and often have irregular borders. Dermatologists will look at the pigment pattern with dermoscopy to evaluate for change. There is debate about whether these lesions need to be removed. Management is controversial. In most instances, the answer is no since they can be followed over time and their risk of transformation is small. Referral can be helpful to avoid unnecessary surgical removal. There are also certain circumstances when removal is a reasonable option. Reasons to remove nevi include location in hard-to-follow regions such as in the nail, scalp, or in other areas difficult to examination. Removal is reasonable if the nevus is located in sites that are cosmetically unacceptable to the child leading to issues of self-esteem. Removal is indicated of course if a biopsy suggests change or clinically the lesion has changed significantly in color, size, or shape. Patients will trade their congenital nevus for a line scar, which will also grow with the child.

Suggested Readings

Bauer BS, Corcoran J. Treatment of large and giant nevi. *Clin Plast Surg.* 2005;32(1):11-18.

Bett BJ. Large or multiple congenital nevi: occurrence of cutaneous melanoma in 1008 persons. *J Am Acad Dermatol.* 2005;52(5):793-797.

Kinsler VA, Chong WK, Aylett SE, Atherton DJ. Complications of congenital naevi in children: analysis of 16 years experience and clinical practice. *Br J Dermatol.* 2008;159(4):907-914.

Price HN, Schaffer JV. Congenital melanocytic nevi when to worry and how to treat: facts and controversies. *Clin Dermatol.* 2010;28(3):293-302.

Slutsky JB, Barr JM, Femia AN, Marghoob AA. Large congenital melanocytic nevi: associated risks and management considerations. *Semin Cutan Med Surg.* 2010;29(2):79-84.

Tannous ZS, Mihm MC, Sober AJ, Duncan LM. Congenital melanocytic nevi: clinical and histopatholigic features, risk of melanoma, and clinical management. *J Am Acad Dermatol.* 2005;52(2):197-203.

SECTION III

RASHES

How Do You Distinguish Serious Systemic Rashes Like Toxic Epidermal Necrolysis and Stevens-Johnson Syndrome From Each Other and From Less Serious Rashes?

Anna S. Salinas, MD and Moise L. Levy, MD

Patients usually appear ill with toxic epidermal necrolysis (TEN) or Stevens-Johnson syndrome (SJS). With either of those conditions, for instance, the skin can be tender when examined. By definition, there will be characteristic involvement of skin and the mucous membranes. Importantly, SJS must be differentiated from other serious skin disorders such as staphylococcal scalded skin syndrome (SSSS) as well as less severe conditions like urticaria.

Differentiating Staphylococcal Scalded Skin Syndrome From Stevens-Johnson Syndrome/ Toxic Epidermal Necrolysis

Staphylococcal scalded skin syndrome (SSSS) is an infectious disease caused by a localized staphylococcal infection, which then releases an exfoliative toxin. The toxin causes cleavage within the upper layers of the epidermis that results in peeling by disrupting a molecule called desmoglein 1 that helps keep skin cells attached to each other. The main clinical differentiator is that SSSS by definition does not affect the mucous membranes. In the mucous membranes, there is enough of a redundant molecule called desmoglein 3 to protect the mucous membranes from cleavage by the exfoliative toxin. If the diagnosis is in question, a biopsy with frozen section analysis can help to differentiate SJS and TEN (which both are characterized by full thickness epidermal necrosis) from SSSS (which

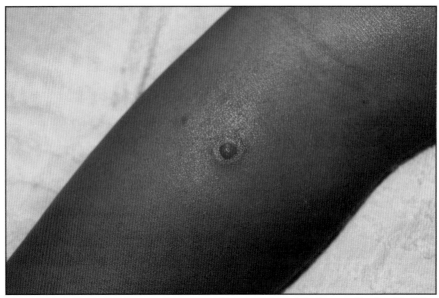

Figure 14-1. Target lesion on the arm with central vesicle in a patient with SJS.

demonstrates a split in the superficial epidermis). Therefore, if there are no lesions in the mouth and the sclerae are white and unaffected, SSSS is much more likely than SJS/TEN.

Another major differentiator is that SSSS typically occurs in children under 5 and especially in neonates, many of whom are not on medications, which can lead to SJS/TEN. Remember in the absence of medications, SJS can still be caused by *Mycoplasma*, which can affect children under 5 years of age.

A third major differentiator is the flexural and neck location of the redness (which often looks like a sunburn) and subsequent peeling in SSSS. SSSS typically is most pronounced in the neck folds, axillae, and inguinal folds.

If a clinical diagnosis is in question, then a biopsy will show the epidermal split in SSSS is very superficial; whereas, in SJS/TEN there is full thickness epidermal necrosis. It is actually very simple to do this rapidly without a biopsy by taking a piece of slough skin and delivering it to an experienced pathologist for a frozen section again to evaluate for degree and depth of epidermal necrosis.

Differentiating Urticaria From Stevens-Johnson Syndrome/Toxic Epidermal Necrolysis

There are several pieces of information from history and physical examination that warrant concern for a diagnosis of SJS/TEN: duration of the lesions for over 24 hours; so-called target or "iris" lesions with fixed dark or erythematous centers (Figure 14-1), vesiculation, or increased skin fragility; occurrence of flulike prodrome; fever; facial swelling; and especially mucosal involvement (Figure 14-2). A history of a new medication being started within 1 to 3 weeks of onset of the eruption is often noted. Urticaria, however, is generally an evanescent eruption. The individual skin lesions—papules or

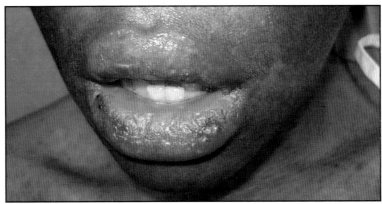

Figure 14-2. Lips with full thickness necrosis and crusting in patient with SJS.

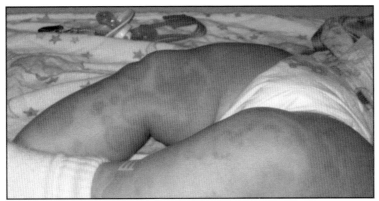

Figure 14-3. Urticarial plaques with clear center in a patient with extensive urticaria due to a virus.

plaques—have lighter centers relative to their periphery (Figure 14-3). Pruritus is often noted as well. These findings are further delineated in Table 14-1. It is imperative that if any feature suggestive of SJS/TEN is found to be present, the patient be closely monitored for the possible development of SJS/TEN and further work-up, including a skin biopsy, be considered.

Pathogenesis of Stevens-Johnson Syndrome/ Toxic Epidermal Necrolysis

There are a multitude of presumed causes for SJS, TEN, and urticaria ranging from medications, to malignancies, to infectious etiologies. Many of these causes overlap among these diagnoses, with medications (especially penicillins, sulfonamides, other antimicrobials, and anticonvulsants) representing the most common culprits for both SJS/TEN and urticaria. Furthermore, for urticaria and SJS/TEN, often the causative agent may be unknown. It is worth mentioning, however, that while the more serious TEN is

Table 14-1

Distinguishing Steven-Johnson Syndrome and Toxic Epidermal Necrolysis From Urticaria

	Steven-Johnson Syndrome/ Toxic Epidermal Necrolysis	*Urticaria*
Prodrome	Flulike symptoms lasting 1 to 14 days: fever, malaise, headache, cough, sore throat	Not typically described, although many episodes of urticaria in children are caused by a typical upper respiratory infection
Clinical findings	Erythematous macules or patches with central necrosis, vesicles, bullae often starting on the face, upper trunk, and extremities Areas of denudation; petechiae, purpura Lesions may be targetoid or may not be well demarcated Diffuse erythema may be present and this skin is at risk for necrosis	Large wheals Erythematous plaques Diffuse, confluent erythema not typically seen
Nikolsky sign (lateral pressure on skin will cause blistering or sloughing)	Positive	Negative
Pain at site of skin involvement	Early in course, pain out of proportion to physical findings Burning or paresthesias may be present	"Burning" may be described, however, pruritis is prominent; pain should not be a predominant feature
Location	Widespread involvement Initially manifests on face, upper trunk	May be widespread as well, distribution is variable Commonly seen on extremities, torso
Natural history	Rapid progression of lesions, with development of vesicles and bullae that then rupture	Individual wheals rapidly develop and regress in 12 to 24 hours In chronic urticaria, hives will be present most days of the week for 6 weeks or longer
Mucosal involvement	Two or more distinct sites of mucosal involvement, ocular, oral, genital Painful crusts and erosions may occur over affected mucosal sites	Not typically described

(continued)

Table 14-1 (continued)
Distinguishing Steven-Johnson Syndrome and Toxic Epidermal Necrolysis From Urticaria

	Steven-Johnson Syndrome/ Toxic Epidermal Necrolysis	*Urticaria*
Ocular involvement	May have severe purulent conjunctivitis, photophobia, and/ or conjunctival itching or burning	No
Signs of systemic involvement	Urethritis resulting in dysuria or urinary retention	Not typically described
Histopathological findings	Early: Perivascular mononuclear cells (usually T-lymphocytes) with epidermal keratinocyte necrosis. Late: Subepidermal vesiculation with epidermal necrosis	Typically with minimal findings; may see dermal edema, vascular dilatation, mild perivascular infiltrate predominantly consisting of monocytes and lymphocytes

invariably attributed to medications, SJS may be attributed to either drugs or infection, and recent studies have shown that the infections most commonly implicated in pediatric SJS/TEN include *Mycoplasma pneumoniae* and herpes simplex virus (more commonly implicated in erythema multiforme than SJS). Many cases of SJS due to *Mycoplasma* are atypical in that there is more mucosal than cutaneous involvement.

Once the diagnosis of SJS or TEN is made, distinguishing between SJS and TEN is relatively straightforward, as it is based solely on the body surface area (BSA) affected, with SJS manifesting involvement of less than 10% of BSA and TEN involving over 30% of BSA. The diagnosis of "SJS/TEN overlap" is often used for those individuals with between 10% and 30% of body surface sloughing.

Therapy for SJS and TEN is controversial but all of the possible offending medications and their cross-reactors should be stopped immediately. Supportive care with special attention to fluid and electrolyte status, pain control, and monitoring for infection as well as wound care with plain petrolatum gauze are essential. Historically, systemic steroids have been used for SJS and TEN but there may be an increased risk of infection from the immunosuppressing effects of steroids especially in patients with large body surface areas involved. More recently intravenous immunoglobulin (IVIG) has been used with many reports showing decreased morbidity and mortality especially in TEN and especially when IVIG is started early in the course.

Suggested Readings

Bastuji-Garin S, Rzany B, Stern RS, Shear NH, Naldi L, Roujeau JC. Clinical classification of cases of toxic epidermal necrolysis, Stevens-Johnson syndrome, and erythema multiforme. *Arch Dermatol.* 1993;129(1):92-96.

Forman R, Koren G, Shear NH. Erythema multiforme, Stevens-Johnson syndrome and toxic epidermal necrolysis in children: a review of 10 years' experience. *Drug Safety.* 2002;25(13):965-972.

Mockenhaupt M, Viboud C, Dunant A, et al. Stevens-Johnson syndrome and toxic epidermal necrolysis: assessment of medication risks with emphasis on recently marketed drugs. The EuroSCAR-Study. *J Invest Dermatol.* 2008; 128(1):35-44.

Nirken MH, High WA. Stevens-Johnson syndrome and toxic epidermal necrolysis: clinical manifestations; pathogenesis; and diagnosis. In: Basow DS, Levy ML, eds. *UpToDate.* Waltham, MA: UpToDate; 2011.

Ravin KA, Rapparport LA, Zuckerbraun NS, Wadowsky RM, Wald ER, Michaels MM. *Mycoplasma pneumoniae* and atypical Stevens-Johnson syndrome: a case series. *Pediatrics.* 2007;119(4):e1002-1005.

Roujeau J-C. Clinical heterogeneity of drug hypersensitivity. *Toxicology.* 2005;209:123-129.

Saini S. Chronic urticaria: Diagnosis, theories of pathogenesis, and natural history. In: Basow DS, ed. *UpToDate.* Waltham, MA: UpToDate; 2011.

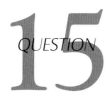

15

WHEN SHOULD I REFER RECURRENT ORAL ULCERS TO A SPECIALIST?

Bhavik S. Desai, DMD, PhD; Andres Pinto, DMD, MPH, FDS RCSEd; and Faizan Alawi, DDS

Oral ulcerations can arise from a variety of different etiologies. Trauma is the most common cause of mouth ulcers in the pediatric patient; accidental mucosal bites, fractured teeth, and orthodontic hardware are frequent sources. However, oral ulcers may also arise from an array of other local or systemic conditions. These include inflammatory and autoimmune disorders, infectious agents, nutritional deficiencies, blood dyscrasias, and malignancy. Importantly, most oral ulcerations do not have any distinctive clinical features. Thus, tissue biopsies are often required to determine the underlying cause of the ulceration, especially in cases of persistent or recurrent lesions. However, most ulcers also exhibit nonspecific histology. Thus, the clinician will often require additional information, including blood or serological testing, to make an appropriate clinical diagnosis. Ultimately, if the root source of the ulceration is not identified, the lesions may persist or recur with relative frequency. This can prove to be a significant challenge to treatment and often results in referral of these patients to specialized practitioners, including dental practitioners, for further evaluation and management. Below, we highlight several conditions that are commonly associated with multifocal, recurrent, or nonhealing oral ulcerations. Familiarity with these disorders will aid the practitioner in the decision-making process for a given patient with oral ulcers.

Traumatic Ulcers

Traumatic ulcers are typically solitary, self-limiting, and usually resolve within days of the injury. Unless the trauma persists, these lesions tend not to recur. Indeed, recurrent or persistent traumatic ulcers in a child's mouth should raise the suspicion of chronic habits such as lip or cheek biting or parafunctional habits involving sharp objects. Riga-Fede disease is an ulceration that results from repetitive trauma to the ventral tongue or the lingual frenulum by either natal teeth or erupting teeth in neonates and toddlers.[1]

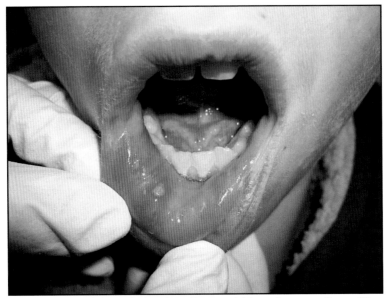

Figure 15-1. Aphthous lesion in a 9-year-old female presenting with a history of recurrent painful mucosal ulcers.

Recurrent Aphthous Stomatitis

Recurrent aphthous stomatitis (RAS) ("canker sores") is the second most common cause of oral ulceration. Lesions are classified as minor, major, and herpetiform based on their clinical appearance. Unlike recurrent intraoral herpes (see below), RAS usually develops on nonkeratinized mucosa (Figure 15-1). This includes all oral mucosal surfaces except the dorsum tongue, attached gingiva (gingival tissues immediately proximal to the teeth), and hard palate; the herpetiform variant can affect any mucosal surface. While RAS is often a self-limiting condition, recurrences are not uncommon. In addition, RAS or RAS-like lesions are often observed in association with systemic disturbances, including nutritional and hematologic deficiencies, autoimmune processes, and gastrointestinal (GI) inflammatory conditions.[2] Thus, if the aphthous lesions have a propensity for multifocality, frequent recurrence, or persistence, laboratory investigation may be required to determine the underlying etiology. When needed, treatment usually consists of topical corticosteroid therapy; systemic therapy may be needed in refractory or severe cases.

Ulcerations Associated With Viral Infection

Viral infections, including those caused by herpes simplex (primary herpetic gingivostomatitis) and Coxsackie A (herpangina), are typically associated with the acute onset of mucosal vesicles that rupture and ulcerate. Various constitutional signs and symptoms usually precede the development of the oral lesions. These may include fever, malaise, tender cervical lymphadenopathy, and fatigue. While the oral manifestations may be dramatic, spontaneous resolution within 7 to 14 days is the norm. Palliative therapy is

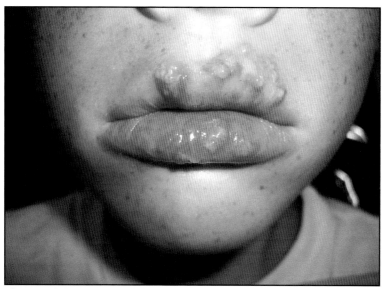

Figure 15-2. Recurrent labial and perioral HSV infection in an 8-year-old child. The gingiva and intraoral mucosae were spared.

often necessary, but no additional therapeutic intervention is typically warranted. In contrast, pediatric human immunodeficiency virus (HIV) infection or other immunodeficiency can manifest with florid oral ulcerations, which are often persistent. Unfortunately, antiretroviral therapies targeted against HIV are often associated with their own significant complications, including oral ulceration.[1]

RECURRENT (SECONDARY) HERPES

Recurrent oral herpetic lesions classically develop on the lips (Figure 15-2) or intraoral keratinized tissues, including the hard palate and attached gingiva. Onset may be characterized by prodromal symptoms like fever, malaise, and irritability. Importantly, herpetic lesions are often self-limiting and do not require therapy. However, in some patients, these ulcerations may recur frequently or cyclically, especially in peripubertal or postpubertal adolescents. In immunosuppressed patients, recurrent herpes may develop on any mucosal surface or persist for extended periods of time, thereby making an empiric diagnosis more challenging.[3] In these latter scenarios, diagnostic testing for herpes such a cytologic smear, direct fluorescence antibody, tissue biopsy, culture, or polymerase chain reaction may be warranted. Antiviral therapy, including prophylactic usage, may help accelerate healing or pre-empt lesion development. We typically recommend prophylactic therapy in patients who report five or more recurrences in 1 year.

Erosive, Vesiculoerosive, and Autoimmune Conditions

Many of the classic autoimmune vesiculobullous diseases, including mucous membrane pemphigoid and pemphigus vulgaris, only rarely affect the pediatric population. In contrast, less common conditions, including linear immunoglobulin A disease, have a propensity for childhood onset. Irrespective of the disease, these disorders are characterized by the development of diffuse vesicles and bullae that rupture and ulcerate. The ulcerations may coalesce to produce large areas of erosion.[1] A tissue biopsy is required for accurate diagnosis. Treatment will depend on the extent of mucosal and possible cutaneous involvement.

ERYTHEMA MULTIFORME

This is an unusual, hypersensitivity-type reaction that develops in response to infectious, chemical, or drug triggers.[4] Mucocutaneous findings are typical. However, we have encountered a number of cases in which erythema multiforme (EM) was restricted to the mucosa. Hemorrhagic crusting of the lips is characteristic. The intraoral lesions initially develop as diffuse vesicles and bullae and eventuate as ulcers. Temporal association with a recent illness or consumption of a new medication and abrupt onset of the mucosal lesions may assist in the diagnosis of this condition. Although nonspecific, a tissue biopsy may help in eliminating other sources of ulceration. Systemic steroid therapy is typically necessary. Recurrent EM is often associated with reactivation of the herpes simplex virus. Thus, prophylactic antiviral therapy may also be beneficial. If the trigger is thought to be a drug, elimination of the offending medication is required.

LICHEN PLANUS, LICHENOID MUCOSITIS, AND ALLERGIC STOMATITIS

These conditions are all characterized by an immune-mediated reaction that may be restricted to the oral mucous membranes. While a relatively common occurrence in adult patients, these conditions are less common in the pediatric population.[5] Nonetheless, the clinical appearance of the lesions and their associated triggers are common to all ages. Common culprits include chronic exposure to flavoring agents, including cinnamaldehyde (cinnamon), medication-related hypersensitivity, and contact reactions to dental materials. However, in many instances, the underlying trigger cannot be identified. Oral lesions typically manifest as irregularly shaped ulcerations, erythematous, or white mucosal plaques (Figure 15-3), which may be accompanied by radiating white striae or as desquamative gingival lesions. Tissue biopsy is needed for appropriate diagnosis. Depending on the extent and severity of disease, topical or systemic corticosteroids are required for effective resolution. In cases where a possible trigger has been identified, elimination of the agent is usually required to ensure appropriate therapeutic response and minimize recurrence. Chronic graft-versus-host disease (GVHD) often mimics the clinical and histologic appearance of lichenoid lesions. Hence a history of allogeneic bone marrow transplant should significantly increase the index of suspicion for GVHD.

Ulcerations Associated With Systemic Disease

Mouth ulcers that arise in association with systemic disease have a tendency to be persistent, multifocal, or exhibit frequent recurrence. In cases where the oral lesions are temporally associated with the development of cutaneous or systemic findings, diagnosis,

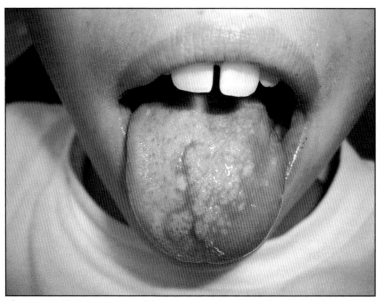

Figure 15-3. Seven-year-old male complaining of painful dorsal and left tongue, clinically consistent with lichen planus.

and appropriate treatment of the extra-oral disease may lead to resolution of the oral ulcerations. Conversely, oral ulcers may be among the earliest clinical manifestations of systemic disease and precede the development of dermatologic or systemic complications by weeks, months, and sometimes, years. These are the patients that typically present to primary care clinicians and for whom referral may be warranted. Similarly, a strong case for referral can be made in cases of long-standing oral ulcers that have failed to respond to topical or systemic corticosteroids.

Behçet Disease

This chronic, inflammatory disorder is characterized by a clinical triad of RAS, recurring genital ulcers, and ocular inflammation. Oral ulcers are more common in children than uveitis. MAGIC (**m**outh **a**nd **g**enital ulcers with **i**nflamed **c**artilage) syndrome is a variant of Behçet disease characterized by RAS, genital ulcers, and chondritis.[2] Laboratory findings are not typically helpful in making a clinical diagnosis of Behçet disease. However, it is important to rule out infectious etiology or granulomatous inflammatory processes, including Crohn's disease. Afflicted patients typically require systemic therapies.

Gastrointestinal Disorders

Crohn's disease and ulcerative colitis are the most common inflammatory bowel diseases. Celiac disease adversely affects the mucosa of small bowel and results from sensitivity to gluten. Evidence suggests that celiac disease is an autoimmune disorder. Persistent or recurrent RAS-like oral ulcers are commonly encountered in Crohn's disease, ulcerative colitis, and celiac disease. In addition, nonspecific erythema and diffuse mucosal erosion may be

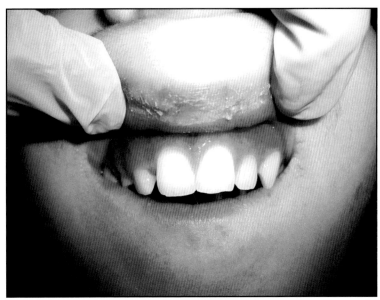

Figure 15-4. Gingival edema, erythema, and erosion in a 7-year-old male complaining of GI distress subsequently diagnosed as ulcerative colitis.

seen (Figure 15-4). Interestingly, Crohn's disease may also be associated with the development of highly characteristic linear ulcerations typically located within the mucobuccal fold. Tissue biopsies of such lesions may reveal granulomatous inflammation.[6] We have encountered several pediatric patients in whom the oral manifestations of Crohn's disease preceded the intestinal disturbances by months, if not years. Association of oral ulcers with a history of GI distress may increase the index of suspicion of a GI disorder. Diagnosis and treatment of the underlying GI disease will often lead to fewer recurrences of oral ulcers.

BLOOD DYSCRASIAS

Neutropenia, lymphopenia, and pancytopenia typically develop in the pediatric population as a result of a genetic predisposition, as a complication of systemic chemotherapy, or secondary to lymphoreticular malignancies. In general, these patients will present with an array of significant systemic complications. Detailed laboratory investigations will often lead to diagnosis. The oral ulcerations are usually nonspecific and may resolve with appropriate therapy. Recurrences are limited by treatment of the underlying dyscrasia.

NUTRITIONAL DEFICIENCIES

Common nutritional deficiencies that cause recurring oral ulcers include iron, folic acid, vitamin B_{12}, and ferritin. In many instances, the ulcers resemble those seen in RAS. In patients with presumed "RAS" that is persistent, widespread, frequently recurrent, or resistant to therapy, laboratory assessment of the aforementioned nutrients should be performed.[7]

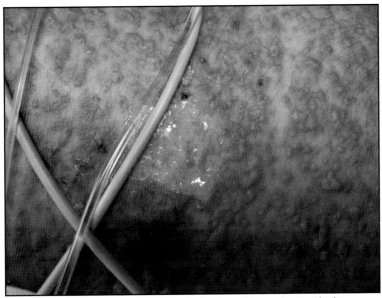

Figure 16-3. Easily denuded skin in toxic epidermal necrolysis.

An appropriate regimen is prednisone or methylprednisolone at 1 to 2 mg/kg/day with a slow taper over 1 to 2 months as liver enzymes are followed. The corticosteroid should be discontinued once the liver enzymes return to normal.

- Arthralgia
  - The presence of arthralgias with an urticarial eruption is suggestive of serum sickness-like reaction (SSLR). SSLR is characterized by polycyclic urticarial wheals with central clearing or purpura. Some people might describe the lesions as urticarial plaques with gray centers. They are common on the trunk, extremities, face, sides of hands, and feet. Unlike drug-induced urticaria, individual lesions are fixed and last days to weeks. Mild oral edema may occur, but no erosions. Patients have high-grade fever and arthralgias. SSLR is commonly triggered by antibiotics that are usually given for 1 to 3 weeks before the reaction occurs. Treatment consists of stopping the offending drug, antihistamines, and supportive care.
- Blisters/erosions
  - When blisters occur, it is always important to consider a diagnosis of Stevens-Johnson syndrome (SJS) or toxic epidermal necrolysis (TEN). SJS and TEN are generally thought to be the same disease but SJS is used when less than 10% body surface area is involved and TEN when greater than 30% body surface area is involved (in between 10% and 30% is SJS/TEN overlap). In order to make a diagnosis of SJS or TEN, 2 or more mucous membranes must be involved. This usually includes the mouth, lips (red, cracked, and often covered with dried blood and erosions on the lingual or buccal mucosa), and the eyes (bilateral conjunctivitis). Anogenital mucosa can also be involved. In some cases of SJS (especially induced by *Mycoplasma pneumoniae*, skin involvement may be absent. However, in classic drug-induced SJS there are targetoid papules and plaques (similar in appearance to erythema multiforme). As the disease progresses, these papules and plaques will blister and form erosions (Figure 16-3). In SJS/TEN, a drug is usually given for 2 to 4 weeks prior

to the reaction developing. Therefore, it is usually antiepileptics, long-term antibiotics, and chronic use of nonsteroidal anti-inflammatory drugs that are the usual culprits. Treatment consists of prompt withdrawal of the drug and administration of intravenous immunoglobulin or cyclosporine in rapidly progressive cases. It is important to provide judicious mouth and skin care. Rinsing with an antiseptic mouthwash is helpful to prevent infection. It is also helpful to apply petrolatum to skin erosions and a nonstick dressing if needed. Antibiotic ointment can be used if there is concern for infection but should not be used empirically due to risk of contact sensitization and systemic absorption through impaired skin barrier. In cases of TEN, electrolytes should also be monitored due to loss of fluids due to the impaired skin barrier.
  - Another condition that can mimic SJS is linear immunoglobulin A (IgA) disease. Linear IgA is characterized by blisters that appear 1 to 13 days after administration of a drug. Vancomycin is a classic offender. Mucous membranes are often not involved, but some cases can mimic SJS as well as other blistering disorders such as bullous pemphigoid or dermatitis herpetiformis. In these cases, a skin biopsy with direct immunofluorescence is helpful in establishing the diagnosis.
- Conjunctivitis
  - Conjunctivitis could be a sign of SJS/TEN when seen with other mucous membrane involvement.
- Mouth sores
  - Mouth sores can be a sign of SJS/TEN when seen with other mucous membrane involvement.
- Phototoxicity
  - Many drugs can cause phototoxic reactions. These occur when a sufficient amount of drug is in the skin and reacts with ultraviolet radiation creating a sunburn reaction. In cases of short-term drug administration (<1 month), this is not a problem. Sun protection should be advised and the drug discontinued if possible. In long-term drug use (months to years), a phototoxic reaction can lead to photodamage and skin cancer. This has recently been observed with the use of voriconazole, an antifungal agent used as long-term fungal prophylaxis and/or treatment in transplant patients or other immunocompromised patients (Figure 16-4).
- Angioedema
  - This is transient edema of the deep dermal, subcutaneous, and submucosal tissues. It is associated with urticaria 50% of the time. It can also be associated with anaphylaxis. One to two cases occur per 1000 new users of angiotensin-converting enzyme inhibitors. The reaction occurs anywhere from 1 day to several years after start of a drug.
- Pustules
  - Acute generalized exanthematous pustulosis is an acute febrile drug eruption with neutrophilia. Clinically and histologically it looks like pustular psoriasis. It is characterized by numerous small, nonfollicular sterile pustules arising within areas of edematous erythema. It starts on the face or intertriginous areas and disseminates over hours. It is seen with antibiotics (B-lactams, macrolides), calcium channel blockers, and others. The time between drug administration and onset of rash is usually less than 2 days. The lesions last 1 to 2 weeks after the drug is discontinued, followed

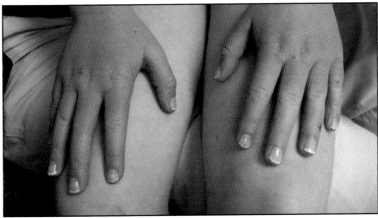

Figure 16-4. Severe phototoxicity of the hands in a voriconazole phototoxic reaction.

by superficial desquamation. Treatment consists of withdrawing the offending drug, topical steroids, and antipyretics.

In all cases, it is always important to take a step back and look at the child. Fever and ill appearance are always worrisome and are consistently seen with the more worrisome drug reactions. When in doubt, a close follow-up appointment is warranted. If two or more mucous membranes are involved, then admission and dermatology consult are indicated. A complete blood count and liver function tests can be very helpful when considering a diagnosis of DRESS syndrome.

Suggested Readings

Koh MJ, Tay Y. Stevens-Johnson syndrome and toxic epidermal necrolysis in Asian children. *J Am Acad Dermatol.* 2009;62(1):54-60.

Segal AR, Doherty KM, Legott J, Zlotoff B. Cutaneous reactions to drugs in children. *Pediatrics.* 2007;120(4): e1082-e1095.

Vinson AE, Dufort EM, Willis MD, Eberson CP, Harwell JI. Drug rash, eosinophilia, and systemic symptoms syndromes: two pediatric cases demonstrating the range of severity in presentation—a case of vancomycin-induced drug hypersensitivity mimicking toxic shock syndrome and a milder case induced by minocycline. *Pediatr Crit Care Med.* 2010;11(4):e38-e43.

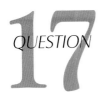

How Do I Treat and Monitor Henoch Schönlein Purpura?

Leslie Castelo-Soccio, MD, PhD

Henoch Schönlein purpura (HSP) is small vessel vasculitis that can affect the skin, gastrointestinal tract, kidneys, joints, and, rarely, the lungs and central nervous system. It is the most common vasculitis in children. HSP is typically diagnosed by the characteristic papular purpuric rash of vasculitis and associated symptoms. The prodrome is typically fever, headaches, and anorexia followed by the rash that occurs in 100% of patients. Fifty percent of patients have the rash as their presenting sign. The typical rash is composed of red macules and papules, which progress to purple papules and plaques. The initial presentation can also be with petechiae or hemorrhagic vesicles, which can be confused with disseminated meningococcal disease or rocky mountain spotted fever (Figures 17-1 and 17-2). HSP can also present with urticarial lesions but they are more purpuric than typical urticaria and not evanescent. Urticarial lesions of HSP are still localized to dependent areas such as legs and may progress to typical palpable purpura over the course of a few days. Various stages of the eruption are usually present simultaneously. The lesions may blanch initially, but they progress to palpable purpura as they mature. The rash usually occurs in dependent areas, including the legs, buttocks, perineum, and lower abdomen but can also appear on other parts of the body, such as the elbows, arms, face, and trunk. Children younger than 2 more frequently have involvement of the head and upper extremities in addition to the typical areas.

Most children with HSP (75%) have joint pain and swelling that most commonly affects large joints, such as the knees, ankles, and elbows, although the hands and feet can be affected. The arthritis usually resolves over several days. Stomach pain is intermittent and extremely common (85% of patients with HSP) and typically is accompanied by nausea, vomiting, or diarrhea but may be a symptom of intussusception. Intussusception can also be the presentation of HSP as can scrotal edema mimicking testicular torsion. Kidney involvement occurs in a smaller proportion of patients (30% to 50%); however, it can present up to 6 months after the start of the illness. Renal involvement includes mild hematuria or proteinuria but also sometimes manifests as oliguria and renal failure. Permanent kidney damage is seen in 20% of patients that develop nephrotic or nephritic syndrome.

Figure 17-1. Henoch Schönlein purpura on the lower extremities of a 13-year-old male manifesting as hemorrhagic vesicles in addition to purpura.

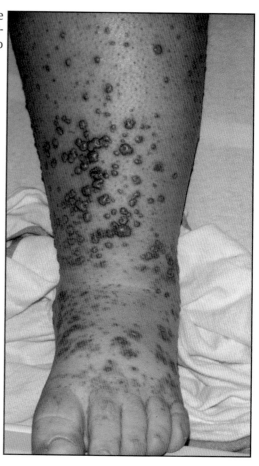

Figure 17-2. Henoch Schönlein purpura located on the upper extremity in a 13-year-old male.

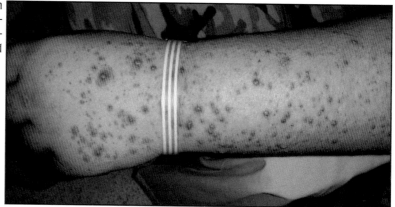

HSP primarily affects children although it can be seen in adults. In children, it is more common in males (2:1 males to females). The median age is 5 years with 75% of cases occurring in children 2 to 11 years of age. Upper respiratory infection (most commonly Group A *streptococcus*) precedes the eruption in 30% to 50% of cases. Many other infections, including *Yersinia*, *Legionella*, parvovirus, adenovirus, *Mycoplasma*, Epstein-Barr virus, and varicella, have also been associated with HSP. Drug-associated HSP has been reported with penicillin, ampicillin, erythromycin, quinine, and quinidine. Vaccines including typhoid, measles, yellow fever, and cholera have also been associated with HSP.

After assessing for alternate causes of the rash and ruling out more serious causes of the presenting symptoms as outlined above, the primary goal is to confirm the diagnosis and to assess for other organ involvement. HSP can be a clinical diagnosis but if in doubt, confirmation of vasculitis is best obtained by a skin biopsy for histology and immunofluorescence to look for immunoglobulin A deposits around blood vessels. It is important to note that the severity of the skin disease does not correlate with the severity of internal involvement. Assessment for kidney disease is mandatory as it is typically asymptomatic and can lead to renal failure. Tests to assess for internal involvement include complete blood count (CBC), complete metabolic panel, urinalysis to evaluate for protein and blood, and stool guaiac. Amylase and lipase may be elevated in patients with associated pancreatitis. A CBC usually reveals leukocytosis with a left shift and possibly eosinophilia (if drug is source of HSP). Hemoglobin and hematocrit may be normal or decreased secondary to bleeding. Urinalysis may reveal hematuria, proteinuria, or red cell casts. Antistreptolysin-O titers can be helpful to determine precipitating infection with Group A *streptococcus* in the absence of a culture-proven infection. Tests to assess for alternate causes of leukocytoclastic vasculitis include a hepatitis-screening panel, antinuclear antibody test, antineutrophilic cytoplasmic antibodies, rheumatoid factor, complement levels, and cryofibrinogens and cryoglobulins. If the history of antecedent infection and symptoms is consistent with HSP, these extensive tests for alternate causes are usually not necessary.

Imaging of the scrotum by ultrasound may be necessary if scrotal edema is a presenting sign in order to rule out testicular torsion. Alternatively, if severe abdominal pain is the presenting sign, then intussusception should be ruled out.

The need to treat HSP depends on the severity of other organ involvement. Admission to the hospital is indicated if needed to control abdominal pain, aid in electrolyte repletion for severe or protracted vomiting, monitor renal function, or confirmation of the diagnosis. The majority of patients require only supportive care with acetaminophen, elevation of swollen extremities, bland diets and hydration, and homecare. Severe skin or organ disease requiring hospitalization often is treated with 1 to 2 mg/kg of prednisone daily for 1 to 2 months. Duration of treatment is dependent on improvement of organ function on therapy. Early consultation with a nephrologist if there is kidney involvement is important to guide treatment duration. Evidence suggests that early intervention with steroids may be especially helpful for kidney disease and treatment of significant abdominal pain. In children not responding to steroids or who need long-term therapy, azathioprine, methotrexate, and cyclophosphamide can be considered as alternate steroid-sparing agents. Dapsone and colchicines have also been used. Dapsone is particularly helpful in treating purpura and arthralgias. Topical therapy is unnecessary unless areas are blistered. Blistering of the purpuric lesions occurs in a minority of cases but when it occurs, good wound care with topical antibiotics, Vaseline gauze, and protective wraps is essential to prevent infection and diminish discomfort. All unnecessary medications should be discontinued if drug reaction is suspected as the etiology. Patients with renal involvement need special attention to their fluid and electrolyte balance and may need antihypertensive medications. Surgery may be undertaken to treat severe bowel ischemia, and kidney transplant is sometimes necessary to treat patients with severe renal disease resistant to therapy. The majority of patients have self-limited disease and only require supportive care.

Suggested Readings

Bogdanovic R. Henoch Schönlein purpura nephritis in children: risks factors, prevention and treatment. *Acta Paediatr.* 2009;98(12):1182-1889.

Chan KH, Tang WY, Lo KK. Bullous lesions in Henoch Schönlein purpura. *Pediatr Dermatol.* 2007;24(3):325-326.

Chartapisak W, Opastiraskul S, Hodson EM, Willis NS, Craig JC. Interventions for preventing and treating kidney disease in Henoch Schölein Purpura. *Cochrane Database Syst Rev.* 2009;8(3):CD005128.

Den Boer SL, Pasmans SG, Wulffraat NM, Ramakers-VanWoerden NL, Bousema MT. Bullous lesions in Henoch Schönlein Purpura as indication to start systemic prednisone. *Acta Paediatr.* 2010;99(5): 781-783.

Gonzalez LM, Janniger CK, Schwartz RA. Pediatric Henoch Schönlein purpura. *Int J Dermatol.* 2009:48(11): 1157-1165.

McCarthy HJ, Tizard EJ. Clinical practice: diagnosis and management of Henoch Schönlein purpura. *Eur J Pediatr.* 2010;169(6):643-650.

Saulsbury FT. Henoch Schönlein purpura. *Current Opin Rheumatol.* 2010;22(5):598-602.

Weiss PF, Feinstein JA, Luan X, Burnham JM, Feudtner C. Effects of corticosteroid on Henoch Schönlein purpura: a systematic review. *Pediatrics.* 2007;120(5):1079-1087.

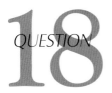

18

HOW DO I DIAGNOSE AND TREAT SCABIES?

Albert C. Yan, MD, FAAP, FAAD

Background

Scabies is a highly pruritic infestation caused by the *Sarcoptes scabei* mite. The organism is contracted through close contact with another infested individual, and manifestations in the skin typically begin within about 1 to 2 months following exposure. The mite feeds on human blood and makes a home for itself by burrowing into the stratum corneum of the skin where the females lay eggs, which hatch to start another cycle of infestation. The infestation is chronic unless treated; however, infestation by canine scabies is typically a self-limited phenomenon since the organism is poorly adapted for infestation of human hosts.

Clinical Manifestations

The infestations can be generalized, but skin findings are most commonly found at warmer body sites and within skin fold areas, such as the web spaces of the fingers and toes; palms; soles; wrists; ankles; axillary, inguinal, and genital sites; inframammary areas; and along the waistline (Figure 18-1). Involvement of the face and scalp are rare except among infants where these areas are more commonly affected. Skin findings include small pink papules, vesicles, pustules, as well as linear or curvilinear pink burrow tracts. These are accompanied by numerous excoriations, since the infestation is often highly pruritic. Some patients who do not scratch as much (as might be seen with neurodevelopmental or psychiatric conditions) may develop heavy infestations. Pink nodules can also be present in patients who develop a hypersensitivity reaction to the infestation. Even after adequate treatment eradicates the mites, this nodular form of scabies can persist for up to 1 year when left untreated.

Secondary bacterial infection can occur if the itching and excoriations are particularly severe and should be treated accordingly when present.

Figure 18-1. Axillary crusted papules and nodules in an infant.

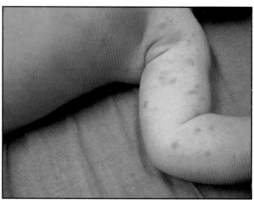

Diagnosis

The diagnosis of scabies can usually be made on clinical grounds. The characteristic presentation of an intensely itchy eruption manifesting with expected skin lesions concentrated at the anatomic sites typical for scabies is often sufficient to make the diagnosis. When scabies is suspected but the findings are less typical, a scraping of intact lesions—ideally, papules, vesicles, and burrows—from higher-yield locations distal to the elbows or the knees (hands, wrists, ankles, and feet) can be performed for diagnostic confirmation. Scraping is traditionally done with a #10 or #15 scalpel blade lubricated with mineral oil. This can be challenging in a moving child, and use of a glass slide or the wooden end of a cotton swab lubricated with mineral oil can be a reasonable substitute. The interdigital webspaces of parents should also be evaluated and if there are typical papules and burrows, it may be easier to scrape a parent if they allow. A negative scraping, however, does not rule out an active scabies infestation, as false-negative scrapings are common. Under microscopy, identification of the mite, the oval translucent eggs, or the tan-brown feces (scybala) is diagnostic for scabies infestation (Figures 18-2 and 18-3). Recently, use of handheld epiluminescence microscopy using polarized light (dermoscopy or dermatoscopy) has been described as a useful, effective, and noninvasive way of confirming the presence of scabies through identification of air bubbles or the triangular pigmented mouthparts of the mite.

Treatment

Permethrin 5% cream remains the mainstay of treatment for scabies infestation in children more than 2 months of age and adults. The cream is applied to the skin from the areas behind the ears down to the toes, with emphasis on applying the cream to intertriginous areas. The cream should be applied to all household members (including those not showing clinical manifestations of infestation) on the same day and left on overnight for about 8 hours before washing off. To treat any new mites arising from hatched eggs, the treatment can be repeated in 7 to 10 days.

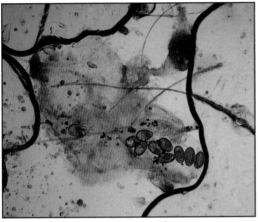

Figure 18-2. Scabies feces and eggs.

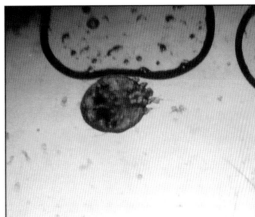

Figure 18-3. Scabies mite.

For infants less than 2 months of age or for pregnant mothers, precipitated sulfur 5% can be extemporaneously compounded into petrolatum for use nightly overnight (8 hours) for 3 nights, washed off each morning, and then repeated about 7 to 10 days later.

Once the initial treatment has been performed, patients will often continue to itch for several days or even a few weeks.

Apparent treatment failures may be explained by the following:

- Incomplete therapy—The patient did not apply the topical agent to all of the recommended areas or left the therapy on for shorter than recommended.
- Scabies resistance to the topical agent—Very uncommon except in those who have been treated on multiple occasions.
- Nodular scabies—A residual hypersensitivity reaction that can persist even after the mites have been eradicated.
- Postscabetic pustulosis—A reactive inflammatory condition characterized by crops of pustules that appear predominantly on the arms, legs, palms, and soles and may spread onto the torso in a cyclical pattern of flares for 5 to 10 days, followed by relative remissions for 2 weeks, and then recurrences. This reaction occurs in the absence of residual live mites. This condition is thought to be related to another clinically similar condition: acropustulosis of infancy.
- Incorrect diagnosis—There are conditions that may mimic a presentation of scabies, and these include atopic dermatitis, dyshidrotic eczema (small vesicles or papules concentrated on the hands or feet or both), Langerhans cell histiocytosis (crusted hemorrhagic papules that may be clustered in the genital areas or scalp, but can be more generalized), dermatitis herpetiformis (a highly itchy skin condition characterized by papules or vesicles on the elbows, knees, buttocks and frequently associated with celiac disease), acropustulosis of infancy (pruritic pustular eruptions on the arms and legs occurring in a cyclical fashion with episodes lasting about 5 to 10 days and occurring every 2 weeks; this condition occurs in infants and toddlers), and bedbug bites (typically in groups and lines of three "breakfast, lunch, and dinner" and typically involving exposed areas or areas covered by loose fitting clothing such as the arms, legs, face, and back; Figure 18-4).

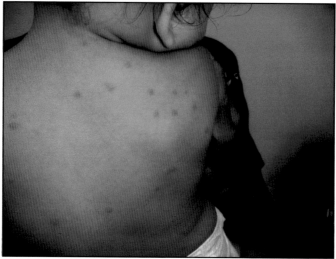

Figure 18-4. Bedbug bites in lines of 3 "breakfast, lunch, and dinner."

For confirmed cases of scabies that have not responded adequately to conventional therapy, oral ivermectin can be used as an off-label therapy for scabies. This is typically given as a single dose and repeated 7 to 10 days later.

Postscabetic itch, postscabetic pustulosis, and nodular scabies can all be treated with topical corticosteroids. Topical triamcinolone 0.025% ointment twice daily to persistently itchy areas for 1 to 2 weeks can be helpful. Oral antihistamines such as diphenhydramine (Benadryl), hydroxyzine (Atarax), cetirizine (Zyrtec), levocetirizine (Xyzal), loratadine (Claritin), desloratadine (Clarinex), and fexofenadine (Allegra) can be given to moderate the symptoms of itch.

Clothing and bedding used within the past 3 days should be washed in hot water and dried in a dryer to eliminate potential fomites. Other clothing or bedding that cannot be washed and dried can be stored in a plastic bag for 1 to 2 weeks.

Suggested Readings

Aterman K, Krause VW, Ross JB. Scabies masquerading as Letterer-Siwe's disease. *Can Med Assoc J.* 1976;115(5): 443-444.

Chulabhorn P, Maliwan D, Sombat S. Sulfur for scabies outbreaks in orphanages. *Pediatr Dermatol.* 2002;19(5): 448-453.

Prins C, Stucki L, French L, Saurat J-H, Braun RP. Dermoscopy for the in vivo detection of *Sarcoptes scabiei. Dermatology.* 2004;208(3):241-243.

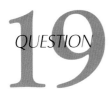

HOW DO I DIFFERENTIATE AND TREAT BUG BITE REACTIONS?

Dirk M. Elston, MD

Background

Bedbugs, spiders, fleas, and mites infest houses and pets, and even groceries harbor biting mites. As a result, the diagnosis and management of bites and stings is a year-round job for the clinician, even in cold climates. Identification of the offending arthropod can be important to eliminate the source of an infestation. When the skin lesions suggest bites, I generally begin the evaluation with a directed history about work, recreation, travel, and pets. Often, the likely source of the bites becomes apparent from the history, but the pattern of the bites or stings can also be helpful in narrowing down the likely culprit (Table 19-1).

Clinical Presentation

Fleabites tend to be papulovesicular and cluster on the ankles, lower legs, and forearms where there is exposed skin that the fleas can reach. Often only one child has evidence of fleabites despite flea infestation in the house. This often leads to disbelief from parents about the diagnosis. We often hear the question, "How could my child have fleabites if no one else is being bitten?"

Chigger bites tend to be papular, often with a central punctum or excoriation and frequently with a peripheral vascular steal phenomenon, causing a pale blanching of the skin surrounding the zone of erythema. They tend to cluster on the ankles (Figure 19-1), at the sock and underwear lines, and on the penis and scrotum in males. These areas are at highest risk for chigger bites because they are exposed when walking through or sitting in the grass and weeds where the chiggers live.

Fire ant stings begin as painful urticarial lesions that evolve to intensely itchy erythematous papules and pustules (Figure 19-2). The fire ant grips the skin with its jaws and pivots, creating multiple stings. This results in recognizable rosettes (Figure 19-3).

Table 19-1

Typical Location and Pattern of Various Types of Bites

Arthropod	Morphology of Bite	Distribution
Flea	Papulovesicular	Ankles, lower legs, and forearms
Chigger	Papular, often with a central punctum or excoriation	Sock and underwear lines, on the penis and scrotum in males
Fire ant	Rosette of pustules	Legs most common
Bedbugs	Wheals or papules in a row	Exposed skin

Figure 19-1. Chigger bites.

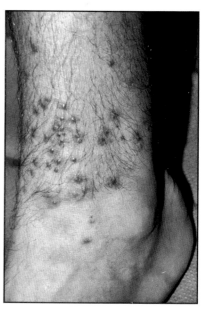

Figure 19-2. Pustular phase of fire ant stings.

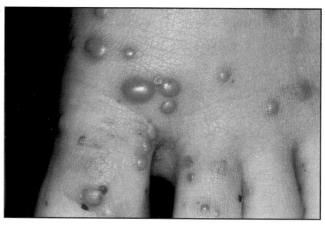

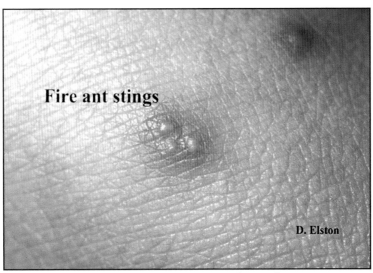

Figure 19-3. Characteristic rosette of stings from a fire ant.

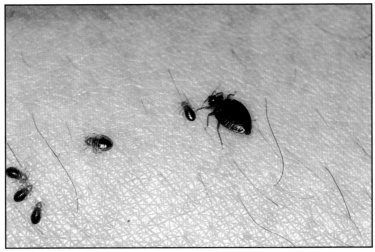

Figure 19-4. Bedbugs.

Bedbugs (Figure 19-4) typically crawl along exposed skin, delivering a series of bites (breakfast, lunch, and dinner), but this pattern is not pathognomonic. When bedbugs are suspected, the linens should be examined just before sunrise, and the mattress, headboard, cracks, and crevices should be inspected for nit-like eggs and bloody feces. Trained dogs have recently been used to detect bedbug infestation.

Mosquito bites begin with urticarial wheals that evolve to intensely pruritic papules. Biting flies generally produce a painful wheal. Spider bites are typically painful and necrotic. Black widow bites produce acute abdominal symptoms that overshadow the local cutaneous reaction. Brown recluse spiders produce dermonecrotic reactions that can be quite extensive.

Special populations of patients develop more exaggerated responses. Atopic individuals develop more prominent papular urticaria from a variety of bites. Those with

Figure 19-5. Annular hypersensitivity reaction simulating erythema migrans.

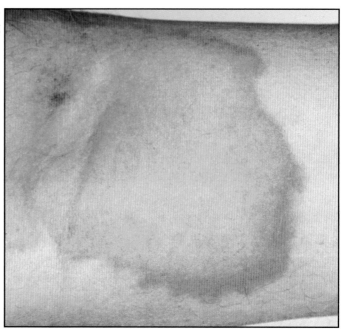

repeated exposure to a biting insect may develop anergy, but often develop severe annular hypersensitivity reactions that may be mistaken for erythema migrans of Lyme disease (Figure 19-5). Patients with HIV infection may demonstrate a recall phenomenon with reappearance of old bite reactions. This may occur in patients with hematopoietic malignancies as well.

Therapy

Most bite reactions can be managed with topical antipruritics, such as camphor and menthol lotion, or topical anesthetics such as lidocaine and pramoxine. More persistent reactions typically respond to topical corticosteroids. I usually use desonide cream or lotion in children, although more severe reactions may require application of triamcinolone 0.1%, fluocinonide 0.05%, or even clobetasol 0.05% in cream or ointment form (in older children). The appropriate strength is based on the severity of the reaction, with fluorinated steroids reserved for lesions on the trunk and extremities. Nodular reactions can be treated with corticosteroid under occlusion, although this increases the risk of atrophy, especially with more potent corticosteroids. Antihistamines can reduce the initial wheal and flare reaction but have no effect on chronic bite or sting reactions. Their only place in the management of chronic reactions is to produce drowsiness, allowing the patient (and the parents) to get some sleep. This can also be accomplished through the use of topical antipruritics and anesthetics.

Arthropod reactions are typically intensely pruritic and often drive patients to despair. I see quite a few patients who beg me to excise chronic bite reactions to relieve the unrelenting pruritus. This is seldom necessary, as refractory reactions usually respond quite well to intralesional injections of triamcinolone in concentrations of 2.5 to 10 mg/mL. The injection is delivered into the heart of each lesion, causing the lesion to blanch.

Avoid more superficial or deeper injections, as these are more likely to produce atrophy. Atrophy and hypopigmentation are seen with higher concentrations of corticosteroid and may extend outward along lymphatic channels.

Flea treatments for animals should be prescribed by a veterinarian, and these include fipronil, imidacloprid, nitenpyram, and selamectin. Pets with areas of hair loss, dermatitis, or dandruff, in patches or preferentially affecting the head or rear quarters, should be evaluated by a veterinarian for flea, *Cheyletiella*, or other mite infestation.

Bee and vespid stings can cause exaggerated local reactions, as well as anaphylaxis. Those who experience anaphylactic reactions should carry epinephrine and should be instructed in the use of the autoinjector before they leave the office. After using an auto-injector, the patient should be evaluated in an emergency department. Approximately 35% of patients with vespid reactions seen in the emergency department for systemic reactions to stings require epinephrine, and approximately 16% require more than a single dose. Even in the absence of anaphylaxis, stings can trigger important systemic manifestations, including arrhythmia, myoglobinuria, or hemoglobinuria with acute tubular necrosis. Desensitization improves quality of life for children with severe bee and vespid allergy, so these children should be referred to an allergist. Anaphylaxis to stings can also be a presenting sign of underlying mastocytosis, so a cutaneous examination should be performed and a mast cell tryptase evaluation is reasonable.

Prevention

Insect repellents remain useful, with picaridin gaining market share, but *N,N*-diethyl-meta-toluamide (DEET) still in widespread use. The American Academy of Pediatrics recommends limiting the concentration of DEET used on children and notes a plateau of efficacy at 30%. Many formulations with lower percentages are available. A soybean oil formulation (Bite Blocker for Kids, HOMS, Pittsboro, NC) also performed reasonably well in an arm box study, providing roughly 90 minutes of protection against mosquito bites. Permethrin-treated clothing is effective against chigger and tick bites. Control of standing water, mosquito traps, community spraying programs, and stocking of ponds with fish to consume mosquito larvae also play an important role in preventing bites.

Suggested Readings

Chippaux JP, Stock RP, Massougbodji A. Methodology of clinical studies dealing with the treatment of envenomation. *Toxicon*. 2010;55(7):1195-1212.

Dryden MW. Flea and tick control in the 21st century: challenges and opportunities. *Vet Dermatol*. 2009;20(5-6):435-440.

Elston DM, Do H. What's eating you? Cat flea (Ctenocephalides felis), part 2: prevention and control. *Cutis*. 2010;85(6):283-285.

Rudders SA, Banerji A, Katzman DP, Clark S, Camargo CA Jr. Multiple epinephrine doses for stinging insect hypersensitivity reactions treated in the emergency department. *Ann Allergy Asthma Immunol*. 2010;105(1):85-93.

The images were produced while the author was a full-time federal employee. They are in the public domain.

WHAT ARE THE KEYS TO RECOGNIZING THE RASH OF LUPUS, DERMATOMYOSITIS, AND JUVENILE IDIOPATHIC ARTHRITIS?

Andrea L. Zaenglein, MD

The cutaneous manifestations of rheumatic diseases in children can be protean in presentation but there are some useful clues you can use to distinguish them from each other as well as from other childhood rashes.

Systemic Lupus Erythematosus

Systemic lupus erythematosus (SLE) has several distinct presentations in the skin, with three rashes being included in the American College of Rheumatology's (ACR) diagnostic criteria for SLE. These 3 are all made worse by sun exposure. Classically, children with SLE present with arthritis, constitutional symptoms, hematologic disease, and renal disease. These may be accompanied by a malar rash. This erythematous, slightly scaling rash appears over the cheeks and nasal bridge in a classic butterfly-shaped pattern. Discoid skin lesions also appear on the head and neck but can occur elsewhere (Figure 20-1). This rash is more inflammatory, often having active, erythematous borders with central scarring. The malar areas are usually involved as well as the concha of the ears and the scalp. Photosensitivity is the last of the cutaneous diagnostic criteria. Macular erythema on sun-exposed sites in the setting of systemic symptoms should prompt suspicion for a diagnosis of lupus. Other mucocutaneous criteria included in the ACR criteria are alopecia and oral/nasal ulcerations. These findings are fairly rare in children with SLE as compared to adults with the disease. Additional uncommon skin presentations of SLE are listed in Table 20-1. Subacute cutaneous lupus is the skin change seen in neonatal lupus. This form is associated with maternal transfer of Sjögren syndrome A (SSA) (Ro) and Sjögren syndrome B (SSB) (La) (rarely U1RNP) antibodies. The rash is pink-red and often annular, occurring on the head and neck. It can look like tinea corporis or infantile

Figure 20-1. Discoid plaques with dyspigmentation and scarring.

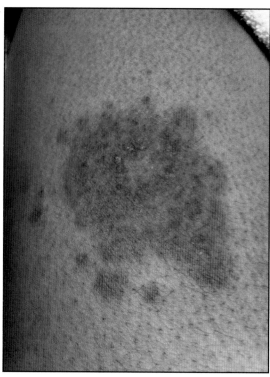

seborrheic dermatitis. Like many of the SLE rashes, it too is photoexacerbated. Babies with neonatal lupus are at risk of complete and partial heart block as well as transient liver and hematologic abnormalities. The rash, however, is usually the last of the findings to appear.

The differential diagnosis of photoexacerbated rashes includes some common viral infections. The "slapped-cheek" rash seen with Parvovirus B19 can recur with sun exposure and can be associated with joint pains and malaise. Epstein-Barr virus too can present with constitutional symptoms and rash, although a typical course is self-limited and easily confirmed by laboratory studies. Several drugs can induce a lupus-like reaction causing fever, arthralgias, and sometimes rash. Minocycline, often used for the treatment of acne, is one of the most common culprits, as well as isoniazid and several anticonvulsants. Tetracyclines, fluoroquinolones, sulfonamides, and nonsteroidal anti-inflammatory agents are medication classes that are known to cause photosensitivity. Nonviral causes of a photoinduced rash include polymorphous light eruption and erythropoietic protoporphyria.

Juvenile Dermatomyositis

Juvenile dermatomyositis (JDM) has several classic features that involve the skin and are often key features in establishing a diagnosis. Rash associated with muscle weakness and elevated muscle enzymes are diagnostic. A heliotrope rash occurs in a mask-like distribution. This rash is typically more pink-purple (violaceous) in color than a classic malar rash seen in SLE. It too is made worse by sun exposure. There is also prominent eyelid involvement and periorbital edema that differentiates it from SLE. Gottron papules

Table 20-1

Cutaneous Presentations of Systemic Lupus Erythematosus, Dermatomyositis, and Juvenile Idiopathic Arthritis

SLE	*Malar Rash*
	Discoid lupus
	Photosensitivity
	Subacute cutaneous lupus
	Lupus profundus
	Livedo reticularis
	Urticarial vasculitis
	Bullous lupus
DM	Heliotrope rash
	Shawl sign
	Gottron sign
	Gottron papules
	Mechanic's hands
	Periungual telangiectasia
	Gingival telangiectasia
	Calcinosis cutis poikiloderma
	Lipodystrophy
JIA	Evanescent rash
	Rheumatoid nodules

are violaceous thin papules or plaques that overlie the knuckles of the hands (Figure 20-2). Similar plaques can localize over the joints of the knees and elbows, often mimicking psoriasis or atopic dermatitis. Also seen are mechanic's hands, a sign of JDM that gives the hands a worn, dry, scaley look. Periungual telangiectasias, as well as gingival telangiectasias, are often observed. These are usually visible with the naked eye but examination with an ophthalmoscope can highlight the dilated capillary loops. Periungual vascular changes can also be used to track disease activity and response to therapy. One characteristic of established JDM that is more commonly seen in children than in adult counterparts is calcinosis cutis. Rock-hard calcified papules or plaques can develop within areas of rash. Ulcerative skin lesions can indicate a systemic vasculopathy and are a sign of aggressive disease. Other long-term sequelae include poikiloderma and lipodystrophy.

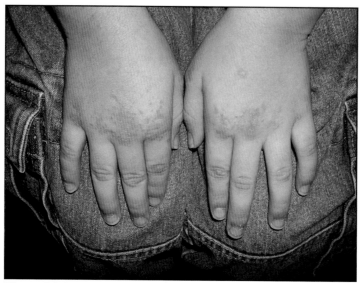

Figure 20-2. Purple papules (Gottron papules) in a patient with dermatomyositis.

Juvenile Idiopathic Arthritis

The evanescent rash of Still disease, encompassed under the revised title of systemic onset juvenile idiopathic arthritis, will classically wax and wane substantially throughout the day. Blotchy, pink macules appear on the trunk and proximal extremities, concentrating in the warmest areas. The rash is not pruritic thus helping to differentiate it from urticaria. The rash is seen in association with daily high fevers and polyarticular arthritis, affecting the knees, ankles, hip, and fingers, with an elevated white count and anemia. Rheumatoid nodules, less common in children with rheumatoid disease, present as rubbery nodules overlying the larger joints of the elbows and knees.

The differential diagnosis of fever with waxing and waning rashes should include urticarial vasculitis, serum sickness-like reaction, acute leukemia, and the autoinflammatory syndromes.

Suggested Readings

Feldman BM, Rider LG, Reed AM, Pachman LM. Juvenile dermatomyositis and other idiopathic inflammatory myopathies of childhood. *Lancet.* 2008;371(9631):2201-2212.

Prince FH, Otten MH, van Suijlekom-Smit LW. Diagnosis and management of juvenile idiopathic arthritis. *BMJ.* 2010; 341:c6434.

Tucker LB. Making the diagnosis of systemic lupus erythematosus in children and adolescents. *Lupus.* 2007;16(8): 546-549.

WHAT CAUSES VULVAR AND PERINEAL ITCHING?

Andrea L. Zaenglein, MD

First off, it is important to closely examine the perineum. Is there redness, scaling, or papular lesions? Is the rash localized to the labia/scrotum, prominent in the creases, or generalized throughout? The appearance and location of the rash (if there is any) can help differentiate the numerous causes of perineal pruritus. Many of the common causes present more frequently in girls, but boys too have their fair share of itching. Table 21-1 lists different clinical presentations and common diagnoses.

Irritant Dermatitis

Undoubtedly, the most frequent cause of perineal itching in preschool to school-aged boys and girls is due to irritation. Irritant dermatitis can be caused by the skin-care products that kids use in the bath and shower. These are often very highly perfumed and contain abundant surfactants to make them lather up nicely. The same goes for bubble bath. As children become more independent in their bathing, they tend to use a lot of soap and do not always rinse off completely. Another common practice that is potentially irritating is the use of wet wipes after toileting. These contain preservatives that are left behind on the skin and can cause an irritant reaction. Also, to put it bluntly, most kids are not the best wipers and they may not be getting bathed frequently enough. Make sure to review hygiene habits and make the necessary product changes for each child. Also review clothing. Children should wear breathable cotton underwear and avoid tight, restrictive pants. In summer, make sure that kids are not sitting in wet swimsuits for long periods, as this too can cause irritation.

Children with atopic dermatitis are also at risk for irritant dermatitis. Avoidance of irritating products is the key to management in these patient as well. Although uncommon, a true allergic contact dermatitis can occur to a wide variety of ingredients in personal-care products. Contact allergy should be considered in refractory cases of perineal dermatitis. Seborrheic dermatitis and psoriasis should also be included in the differential diagnosis of perineal itching with rash. Look for scaling scalp and check for a positive family history.

Table 21-1

Common Causes of Perineal Itching

Description	Location in Groin	Diagnoses to Consider	Hints
Pink-red and scaly	Generalized or localized to labia/scrotum	Irritant dermatitis	Review product usage
		Allergic contact dermatitis	Refractory to treatment
		Atopic dermatitis	Look for eczema elsewhere
Bright red, fairly well-defined plaques	Perianal or in creases	Perianal streptococcal disease	Culture for group A strep
Dull to medium pink, solid, well-defined uniform plaques, +/- scale	Generalized or smaller plaques	Psoriasis	+ Family history, pitted nails, scaling scalp, or plaques elbows/knees
		Seborrheic dermatitis	Look for scaling scalp
Whitish figure 8 pattern with atrophy and petechiae	Labia majora and perianally. In boys, under foreskin	Lichen sclerosus et atrophicus	Ask about constipation, pain with defecating
Pretty clear. Just excoriations	Perianally or throughout	Pinworms	Treat empirically
Irregular, excoriated papules	Throughout perineum	Scabies	Very pruritic
Dry, eczematous patches and plaques with annular borders	Throughout perineum	Tinea cruris	Treat with antifungal first if not sure
Eczematous dry patches studded with firm, pink papules or whitish umbilicated papules	Labia, buttocks, upper thighs	Molluscum contagiosum with eczematous dermatitis	Look for molluscum elsewhere as a clue to diagnosis
Bright red, fairly well-defined plaques	Perianal, intertriginous, glans	Perianal streptococcal disease	Culture to confirm diagnosis

(continued)

Table 21-1 (continued)

Common Causes of Perineal Itching

Description	Location in Groin	Diagnoses to Consider	Hints
Reddish patches with satellite papules and pustules	Perineum and buttocks	Candidiasis	Ask about diaper use
Red, follicular-based papules and pustules	Buttocks most common, perineum and thighs	Staphylococcal folliculitis	Review skin care and hygiene

In any case of perineal itching, no matter the cause, it is important to recommend a sensitive skincare routine. The child should use a gentle, unscented bar cleanser, and liberally use plain petroleum jelly as a protectant. Parents should avoid using bubble baths and scented lotions. Children should use plain toilet paper, avoiding prepackaged wet wipes. Also review proper wiping technique, front to back for the girls. If there is significant redness and irritation, try a low-potency corticosteroid, like 2.5% hydrocortisone ointment, twice daily for a few days to see if there is improvement in symptoms.

One of the most important diagnoses to consider in any girl with vulvar pruritus is lichen sclerosus et atrophicus (LS&A; Figure 21-1). It is not uncommon for girls to go 1 to 2 years without being correctly diagnosed. LS&A begins with erythema that evolves to whitish, atrophic patches. Secondary erosions, fissures, and purpuric changes are characteristic. The affected area typically extends in a figure 8 pattern, from the clitoral hood to the skin surrounding the urethral, vagina, and anal openings. Symptoms of itching are very common. Constipation also results quite frequently. Because the peak occurrence is about 3 to 5 years of age, affected girls can develop some serious issues with constipation. These problems become behavioral and can be quite hard to correct. LS&A is much less common in boys but may be seen especially in the setting of phimosis. Treatment of LS&A consists of short courses of clobetasol ointment and/or topical tacrolimus ointment. Potent topical steroids, such as clobetasol, are often extremely effective. However, their use should be monitored closely for signs of atrophy and potential adrenal insufficiency with overuse. A reasonable approach would be to use clobetasol ointment once to twice daily for 3 to 4 weeks until symptoms are improved then transition to topical tacrolimus daily.

There are also several infectious causes of perineal pruritus to consider. Pinworms, or enterobiasis, are the most common parasitic infection in children. Treatment with mebendazole or other antihelminth is usually done empirically when there is perianal itching without associated rash. Scabies infestation is very pruritic, with irregular, excoriated papules in various stages often seen in the groin. Look for the classic interdigital involvement of the hands. Treat with topical permethrin 5% cream neck to toe overnight. Wash sheets and bedclothes in hot water in the morning. Repeat in 1 week to kill off newly

Figure 21-1. Labia of a young girl showing atrophy (white areas) and hemorrhage typical of lichen sclerosis et atrophicus.

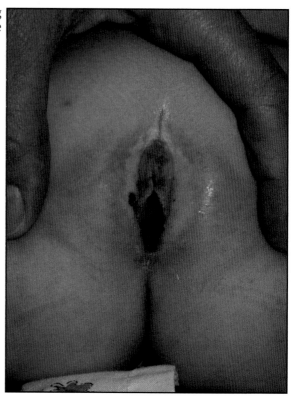

hatched eggs. Tinea cruris is more common in adolescents and young adults but can be seen at any age. Dry, eczematous patches and plaques with annular borders (or even a hint of annularity) are suggestive. When in doubt, treat with an antifungal cream, such as terbinafine, first. This approach will prevent Majocchi granuloma formation (deep follicular infiltration of the fungus necessitating oral antifungal treatment), which can result from inappropriate use of topical steroids. Molluscum contagiosum can induce an eczematous reaction around the classic umbilicated papules that is quite itchy. As treatments for molluscum in the groin are rather limited, controlling the eczematous reaction with a low potency topical corticosteroid ointment and awaiting spontaneous resolution of the molluscum is standard care. Perianal streptococcal disease can occur in the rectal region but also on the glans penis and intertriginous areas. Look for bright red, fairly well-defined plaques. These can wax and wane over several months and spread among family members. Once the infection is confirmed with a culture, an appropriate oral antibiotic, such as amoxicillin, should be given. Topical mupirocin ointment may be used in conjunction as well. But note that recurrences are not unusual. Candidiasis is common in babies still in diapers, due to the moist environment. Consider this diagnosis in older kids who wear nighttime diapers as well. Reddish patches with satellite papules and pustules are characteristic. Treatment consists of a topical antifungal cream, such as clotrimazole, as needed. One of the more common infections seen in younger school-aged children is staphylococcal folliculitis. Red, follicular-based papules and pustules are located mostly on the buttocks but may be seen in the perineum and upper thighs. Often these kids have quite dry skin as well. Make sure to review skin care, moisturize daily, and treat the affected areas with a topical antibiotic ointment, like mupirocin. If deeper abscesses form, consider culture for methicillin-resistant staphylococcus.

Suggested Readings

Fischer G, Rogers M. Vulvar disease in children: a clinical audit of 130 cases. *Pediatr Dermatol.* 2000;17(1):1-6.

Maronn ML, Esterly NB. Constipation as a feature of anogenital lichen sclerosus in children. *Pediatrics.* 2005;115(2): e230-e232. Epub 2005 Jan 3.

Paek SC, Merritt DF, Mallory SB. Pruritus vulvae in prepubertal children. *J Am Acad Dermatol.* 2001;44(5):795-802.

Poindexter G, Morrell DS. Anogenital pruritus: lichen sclerosus in children. *Pediatr Ann.* 2007;36(12):785-791.

WHAT THERAPIES WORK FOR PITYRIASIS ROSEA?

John C. Browning, MD, FAAD, FAAP

Pityriasis rosea (PR) is a common rash seen in children and adults. The underlying cause of PR is unknown but a viral etiology has long been suspected due to clustering of PR in the spring and fall. Human herpesvirus (HHV)-6 and HHV-7 have long been suspected as causative agents of PR but definitive evidence is lacking. One recent study showed the presence of HHV-8 in lesional skin of 7 out of 34 patients with PR. There are also many drugs that can cause a PR-like reaction.

Most patients affected with PR are between the ages of 10 and 35 years, although it has also been reported in infants, younger children, and the elderly. It occurs all over the world without racial or gender predilection.

Most often, PR begins as an erythematous, scaly patch on the trunk known as a herald patch. This patch is usually several centimeters in size and distinctly larger than the rest of the papules and plaques, which make up the eruption (Figure 22-1). Prior to the generalized rash, the herald patch can be mistaken for tinea corporis. A simple potassium hydroxide (KOH) examination or fungal culture can be done to exclude this diagnosis. Lack of history of a herald patch does not exclude PR as some patients will not develop a herald patch prior or may not remember having one, particularly if it was on their back. Several days to weeks after appearance of the herald patch, numerous smaller scaly papules develop on the trunk along the lines of skin cleavage. Because skin cleavage lines run diagonally on the back, this has been described as a "Christmas tree" pattern. The individual papules have a light pink color.

A typical case of PR lasts on average 6 to 8 weeks, although longer and shorter courses have been reported.

When PR affects the face and extremities more than the trunk, it is referred to as inverse PR. This pattern is more common in darker skin types, and postinflammatory hyperpigmentation is common. This hyperpigmentation eventually resolves but may take 6 months or even 1 year to do so. Most patients with PR complain of mild pruritus, although in some cases it may be highly pruritic or asymptomatic.

The differential diagnosis of PR includes pityriasis lichenoides (Figure 22-2), guttate psoriasis, secondary syphilis (Figure 22-3), cutaneous lupus, capillaritis (Figure 22-4), pityriasis versicolor, nummular eczema, and cutaneous T-cell lymphoma.

Figure 22-1. Scaling thin plaques following skin markings in an adolescent boy.

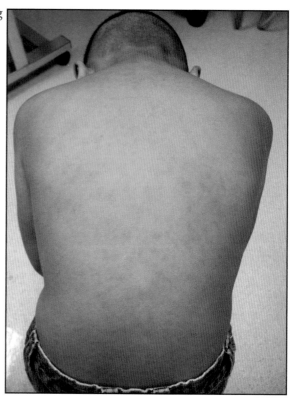

Figure 22-2. Hypopigmented, chronic scaling plaques in a patient with pityriasis lichenoides.

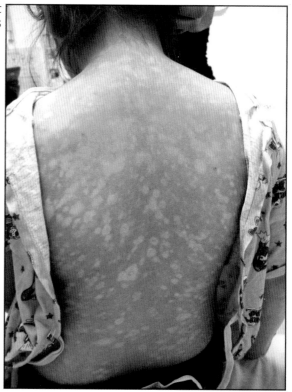

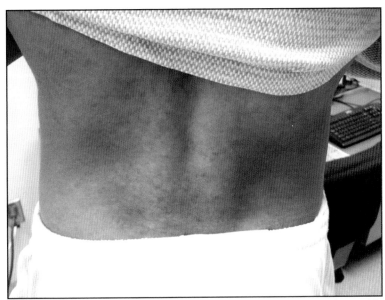

Figure 22-3. Haphazardly oriented scaling papules in a patient with secondary syphilis.

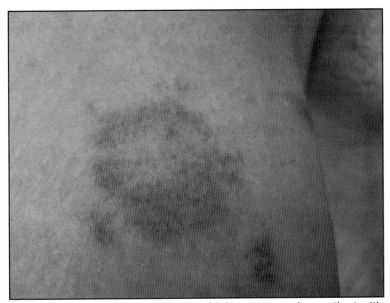

Figure 22-4. Scaling patch with petechial appearance in a patient with capillaritis.

A diagnosis of PR is usually made by history and physical examination alone. In some atypical or long-standing cases, a skin biopsy performed by a dermatologist may prove useful in differentiating PR from other exanthems. Histologic evaluation shows acanthosis with mild psoriasiform hyperplasia and overlying focal parakeratosis.

Treatment for PR is unnecessary since the rash is not contagious and eventually resolves in 1 to 3 months. It is important to remind patients that PR is a benign, self-limited disease, with the exception of potential risks, which may occur during pregnancy. Nonetheless, pruritus or cosmetic concern may prompt requests for treatment. The following treatments may be considered:

- Phototherapy and natural sunlight
  - Narrow-band ultraviolet B phototherapy and natural sunlight have been used successfully in treating PR. Ultraviolet light works by suppressing the cutaneous immune system. A recent report showed low-dose ultraviolet A1 phototherapy in the treatment of PR.
  - During the summer time, a reasonable recommendation for children is moderate daily sun exposure (without burning) to help improve the rash. This can be easily accomplished by daily recreation in a swimming pool, preferably in the morning or late afternoon when the sun's rays are not as strong.
- Oral antibiotics
  - In the past, erythromycin has often been used as a treatment for PR. It has been hypothesized that the anti-inflammatory action of erythromycin, rather than its antibiotic effect, is helpful in resolving PR. New studies, however, have found erythromycin not to be useful in PR and another study did not show any benefit in using azithromycin. A recent study showed a greater benefit in using acyclovir compared to erythromycin in treating PR. Since this is a self-limited process, it is often difficult to tell if the medications are effective or if the disease resolved on its own.
  - In a letter to the editor, one person commented of the effectiveness of clarithromycin in the treatment of PR.
  - There are no published reports of using doxycycline in the treatment of PR.
- Topical steroids
  - Topical steroids offer minimal benefit; they may be helpful when pruritus is present. Use of systemic corticosteroids in PR has not been effective, and the risk of using them is precluded in this benign condition.
- Topical anti-itch products
  - Topical anti-itch products such as those containing menthol or pramoxine have not been studied in PR but may potentially offer a benefit if pruritus is a problem.
  - In other pruritic skin conditions, placement of a moisturizing cream or lotion in the refrigerator can be soothing due to its cooling effects on the skin. Some of this benefit may be due to the cold sensation "distracting" the itch receptors.
- Oral antihistamines
  - Oral antihistamines are not effective in treating PR as the condition is not mediated by histamine.
  - When pruritus is a problem, sedating antihistamines such as diphenhydramine or hydroxyzine may be helpful at night due to their sedative effect.

- Oral acyclovir
  - Recently there has been some evidence that acyclovir may be useful in treating PR. There has also been one report showing development of PR during treatment with acyclovir for another condition, although this could represent a PR-like drug reaction rather than true PR.
  - In vitro studies have shown acyclovir to be ineffective against HHV-6 and HHV-7 and instead have shown ganciclovir and foscarnet to be effective antiviral agents. Presumably this is because HHV-7 lacks the thymidine kinase gene and acyclovir is thymidine kinase dependent. There are no in vivo studies investigating the use of foscarnet or ganciclovir in treating PR. Nephrotoxicity and pancytopenia preclude their use with PR.

Enthusiastic reassurance is indicated as PR resolves with time. Further studies are needed to better understand PR as well as treatment options. Hopefully more definitive treatment will be available in the future.

Suggested Readings

Browning JC. An update on pityriasis rosea and other similar childhood exanthems. *Curr Opin Pediatr.* 2009;21(4): 481-485.

Drago F, Rebora A. Treatments for pityriasis rosea. *Skin Therapy Lett.* 2009;14(3):6-7.

Lim SH, Kim SM, Oh BH, et al. Low-dose ultraviolet A1 phototherapy for treating pityriasis rosea. *Ann Dermatol.* 2009;21(3):230-236.

23

WHAT IS THE APPROACH TO THE NEWBORN WITH BLISTERS?

Kimberly D. Morel, MD, FAAD, FAAP

Blistering in the newborn period may be seen in many medical conditions from a benign, self-limited condition such as a sucking blister to a severe, life-threatening infection, genetically inherited condition, or autoimmune disease. It is important to have an understanding of the differential diagnosis as well as how to differentiate between these various conditions as prompt recognition and treatment of infectious causes of blisters can be life saving. Also, in some cases, blistering may be due to a more chronic condition with associated long-term prognoses.

Although obtaining a medical history is brief in the neonatal period, there are critical facts that should be sought in the maternal history. Review routine laboratory testing performed on the mother during her pregnancy. Be sure your history makes note of maternal history of herpes simplex virus (HSV), syphilis, and other bacterial infections as infections can be acquired both in utero or perinatally. Document gestational age and birth weight as premature infants and lower birth weight infants are at increased risk for infections. Although newborns delivered via cesarean section may have lower risk of spread of vaginal infections, infectious etiologies cannot be excluded, as there can still be ascending spread of infection prior to delivery. Review the timing of onset of blisters and associated symptoms. A pertinent family history should be obtained including any history of skin blistering, skin fragility, nail dystrophy, dental abnormalities, or autoimmune disease. Follow up on the results of newborn screening as rarely metabolic conditions may present with neonatal blistering.

Physical examination should include a thorough evaluation of the morphology and location of the lesions. Note the presence of erosions, pustules, or other lesions present as they may help provide clues to the diagnosis. Presence or absence of erythema around the lesions is also a pertinent finding. Clustered vesicles on an erythematous base located on presenting parts such as the scalp vertex or shoulder classically suggests HSV. A linear assay of blisters may hint at a genodermatosis such as incontinentia pigmenti. Cutaneous erosions without blisters are also an important finding and warrant an evaluation for bacterial, viral, and fungal infection. Be mindful of percent body surface area of blisters and erosions as it may influence fluid and electrolyte balance as well as increase caloric and nutritional requirements.

First and foremost, it is imperative to rule out infection. Although the morphology of the primary lesion may provide a clue to the diagnosis, remember that there may be many overlapping features between infectious and noninfectious causes of blisters and erosions. For example, the eruption of incontinentia pigmenti, usually linear, has been reported to mimic HSV. On the other hand, HSV has been reported to masquerade as mechanobullous disorders. In addition, it is important to consider that any vesicle may involve into a pustule over time and, therefore, this distinction may not always be clinically useful.

The differential diagnosis of the newborn with blisters is broad (Table 23-1). Infectious causes include bacterial infections such as staphylococcal scalded skin syndrome (SSSS), Group B streptococcus, and pseudomonas as well as other important infections such as HSV, varicella, candidiasis (Figure 23-1), and syphilis. Deep fungal infections such as *Aspergillus* have also been reported to present with neonatal vesicles. Severe bullous skin infections with extremely rare viruses have also been reported. When an infectious source is suspected, treatment should be initiated promptly without waiting for results and should be continued even if preliminary cultures are negative if clinical suspicion for infection is high.

Autoimmune blistering disorders present in the neonatal period are due to transplacental transmission of maternal antibodies, even in an asymptomatic mother. Pemphigus vulgaris and pemphigus foliaceus may present in this manner. Epidermolysis bullosa acquisita (EBA) has recently been reported in the neonatal period. Chronic bullous disease of childhood presenting in the newborn is also exceedingly rare. Bullous pemphigoid, generally considered a disease of adults, has been reported in infancy, although most often after 2 months of age. Neonatal lupus may present with vesicular or pseudovesicular lesions as well as widespread erosions in the neonatal period.

Several inherited skin conditions or genodermatoses may present with vesicles in the newborn period. These "blistering" skin conditions include epidermolysis bullosa (EB), Kindler syndrome, epidermolytic ichthyosis (epidermolytic hyperkeratosis), and incontinentia pigmenti. EB is caused by defects in structural proteins involved in the attachment of the epidermis to the deeper skin layers. Kindler syndrome is classified as a subtype of EB. A common history in patients with EB is skin sloughing after a heel stick performed for a newborn screening test or at the site of an adhesive bandage. It is important to note that it is not possible to differentiate subtypes of EB in the newborn period based on physical findings alone. Epidermolytic ichthyosis, a disorder of the keratin proteins in the epidermis, which manifests in childhood and adulthood with thickening of the skin, classically presents in the neonatal period with blisters and erosions. Incontinentia pigmenti is an X-linked dominant condition that often presents in the neonatal period with linear vesicles in a female patient. Aplasia cutis congenita, a condition that may be sporatic or genetically inherited, often presents with erosive lesions in the newborn period. It may also present with a localized bulla within an atrophic plaque.

Cutaneous mastocytosis may present with neonatal blistering. The most common presentation of cutaneous mast cell disease in childhood is that of a solitary mastocytoma. These lesions may urticate when rubbed (called a positive Darier sign) and secondary blistering may potentially occur. Rarely a newborn will present with a diffused form of disease with widespread cutaneous lesions leading to generalized blistering.

Table 23-1

Differential Diagnosis of the Neonate With Blisters

SSSS

HSV

Other infections: Syphilis, Group B streptococcal septicemia, pseudomonas, *Aspergillus*, candida, varicella, other

Cytomegalovirus, Epstein-Barr virus, mycoplasma, chikungunya virus

Autoimmune:

　Transplacental maternal antibodies: pemphigus vulgaris, pemphigus foliaceous, EB acquisita

　Chronic bullous disease of childhood—case report

　Bullous pemphigoid (usually after 2 mo)

　Neonatal lupus erythematosus—can present with widespread erosions

Genodermatoses:

　EB

　Kindler syndrome

　Epidermolytic ichthyosis (previously called epidermolytic hyperkeratosis)

　Incontinentia pigmenti

Zinc deficiency: Bullous acrodermatitis enteropathica

Scabies

Diffuse cutaneous mastocytosis

Congenital erosive and vesicular dermatosis

Congenital self-healing reticulocytosis

Toxic epidermal necrolysis—due to intrauterine graft versus host disease or neonatal gram negative sepsis

Porphyrias

Protein C and S deficiency (hemorrhagic bullae)

Bullous aplasia cutis

Sucking blisters

SSSS indicates staphylococcal scalded skin syndrome; HSV, herpes simplex virus; EB, epidermolysis bullosa

Other notable but rare causes of newborn blistering include toxic epidermal necrolysis. In the neonatal period, this rare but life-threatening condition is due to intrauterine graft versus host disease or neonatal gram-negative sepsis. Porphyrias can present with blisters in the neonatal period classically after phototherapy exposure. Protein C and S deficiencies have been reported to initially present with hemorrhagic bullae in the newborn period. Congenital erosive and vesicular dermatosis is an exceedingly rare condition that presents in the neonatal period with extensive blistering and erosions.

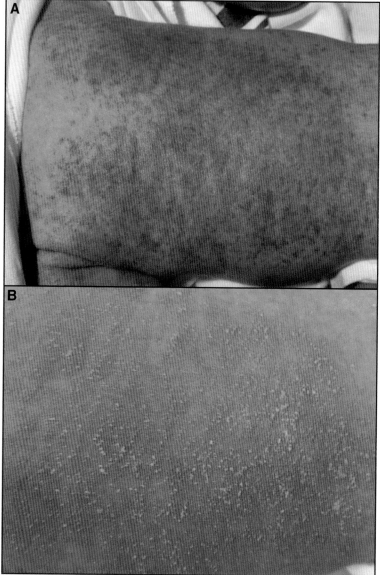

Figure 23-1. Congenital candidiasis (A) 12 hours after birth and (B) at 30 hours when pustules erupted.

Finally, common and benign neonatal conditions should be considered. Sucking blisters usually present in a linear arrangement along the lips or dorsal hand. Although sucking blisters are common in healthy newborns, they may be the presenting sign of other more worrisome conditions such as EB. Erythema toxicum neonatorum usually presents with classic "flea-bitten" erythematous or blanchable red macules usually several days after birth, but may on occasion present with small central vesicles within the lesions. Pustular melanosis (transient neonatal pustular melanosis) presents classically at birth with pustular more than vesicular lesions that resolve within hours to days. Other benign pustular eruptions, which could be confused for vesicles, include milia and sebaceous hyperplasia.

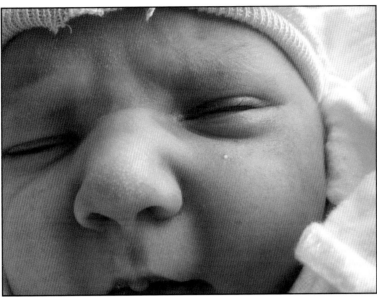

Figure 23-2. Solitary milia on the left upper cheek and sebaceous hyperplasia on the nose and glabella.

Milia present as 1- to 3-mm white noninflammatory papules, and sebaceous hyperplasia presents as pinpoint pustules on the nose and glabella (Figure 23-2). In patients with transient neonatal pustular melanosis the lesions leave behind a hyperpigmented base along with collarettes of scale around the lesions.

After a thorough history and physical examination, laboratory testing is useful to fully evaluate for infection. Cultures, when correctly performed, can aide in obtaining the diagnosis. Samples are best obtained from an intact vesicle or pustule. If no intact lesions are present, then obtain samples from an erosive lesion. Gently cleanse the surface with an alcohol swab and then unroof a blister with a sterile blunt instrument. Swab the blister contents and erosion for a stat gram stain and culture. Swab the base of the unroofed blister for viral culture and rapid direct fluorescent antibody testing for HSV I and II. A Tzanck smear, an additional rapid tool performed mainly by the dermatologist, may reveal multinucleated giant cells in viral infections such as HSV. It is important to note that a negative result does not exclude the diagnosis. SSSS is caused by an exfoliative toxin released from the site of infection. Remember that this site may be distant from the site of blistering or extracutaneous in location, making panculturing the patient important. Fungal and yeast infections may present with erosive lesions especially in preterm infants, and so a swab should be sent to the mycology lab for a potassium hydroxide test for fungal hyphae and culture. Finally, when scabies is suspected, a blunt scraping of the base of a lesion for a mineral oil preparation can be helpful.

Routine histology can be helpful to differentiate certain conditions. Blistering at the level of the stratum granulosum, for example, is supportive of a diagnosis of SSSS. When the diagnosis of EB is suspected, a biopsy of an induced blister performed by a trained provider can be sent for direct immunofluorescence (DIF) testing. Performing a biopsy on a previously formed blister will not yield diagnostic DIF results due to the inflammation that occurs even when a blister may appear to have been of recent onset. Collagen IV is examined to determine the level of split of the blister, and immunofluorescence of proteins collagen VII, type XVII collagen, laminin 332, and integrins attempt to differentiate the subtypes of EB. There is no role for indirect immunofluorescence in the diagnosis of genetically inherited EB.

Diagnosis of autoimmune blistering diseases involves detection of indirect antibodies, usually maternal, by either serology (lupus), enzyme-linked immunosorbent assay, or immunofluorescence (pemphigus, EBA, pemphigoid, and chronic bullous disease of childhood).

- Neonatal lupus is caused by either antibodies to Sjögren syndrome A, Sjögren syndrome B, or U1RNP.
- Pemphigus is caused by antibodies to desmoglein 1 (foliaceus) or desmogleins 1 and 3 (vulgaris).
- EBA is caused by antibodies directed against type VII collagen.
- Chronic bullous disease of childhood is caused most often by antibodies to bullous pemphigoid antigen 2.
- Bullous pemphigoid is caused by antibodies to bullous pemphigoid antigen 1 and/or 2.

Regardless of the cause of the blisters, be aware of topical medication choices, as systemic absorption is likely even upon intact neonatal skin. When skin fragility is present, caution must be taken to assure that nonadherent dressings are chosen to overlie open erosions. Close monitoring of fluid and electrolyte status is important, as there can be significant insensible losses. A gastroenterology/nutrition consultation can help manage the tremendous increase in caloric needs required by neonates with a large body surface area of open erosions. For neonates with EB and mucosal fragility, feeding can be challenging. For bottle-fed infants, use of a Habermann nipple may be helpful and feeding therapy may be required. Pain management is also important, as open erosions can be a source of significant discomfort. Pain control must be balanced with the risk of respiratory depression and oversedation. An oral or nasogastric feeding tube may not be an easy alternative option for increased caloric needs in these patients due to mucosal fragility. In addition, securing lines, tubes, and monitoring can be a challenge as adhesives should not come in contact directly with the skin. The DebRA.org (Dystrophic Epidermolysis Bullosa Research Association of America) Web site as well as the DebRA nurse educator are excellent resources when managing a patient with EB.

Suggested Readings

Eichenfield LF, Frieden IJ, Esterly NB, eds. *Textbook of Neonatal Dermatology.* 2nd ed. Philadelphia, PA: Elsevier Inc; 2008.
Paller AS, Mancini AJ, eds. *Hurwitz Clinical Pediatric Dermatology.* 4th ed. Philadelphia, PA: Elsevier Inc; 2011.

WHAT ARE THE TYPES AND APPEARANCES OF CONTACT DERMATITIS?

Glen H. Crawford, MD and Sharon E. Jacob, MD

The term *contact dermatitis* refers to the skin eruptions that result from external chemical, environmental, and/or mechanical factors. Irritant contact dermatitis (ICD) represents approximately 80% of cases, whereas allergic contact dermatitis (ACD) comprises a significant portion of the remaining 20%, with contact urticaria and protein contact comprising less than 1%. Understanding the salient clinical presentations, causative factors, and treatments for allergic and irritant dermatitis is the focus of this question.

Irritant Contact Dermatitis

ICD is a nonimmunologically mediated inflammatory skin reaction due to damage to the epidermal skin barrier. The most common skin irritants in children are physiologic (such as fecal and urine associated with diaper dermatitis and saliva), with harsh ionic detergent soaps, repetitive exposure to water/wetting, and mechanical friction/trauma also playing a role. As is also seen in the adult population, exposures such as alkalis, metallic salts, alcohol, insecticides, certain plants, dusts, volatile hydrocarbons, and fiberglass may also be seen.

The severity of the reaction will depend on the concentration of the irritating chemical, the site of exposure (such as the sensitive skin of the eyelids), and endogenous factors such as a history of atopic dermatitis and other inflammatory skin conditions (such as psoriasis), which may compromise the epidermal skin barrier function.

Repetitive wetting and drying may lead to ICD in children. So called "lip-licker's dermatitis" is a common eruption in children, with erythema, edema, and fissuring extending from the mucosal lip to beyond the vermillion border (as far as the tongue can reach). Infants also repetitively wet their own faces with saliva as they drool and put their fingers into their mouths. This wetting and drying can lead to an irritant cheek dermatitis that is often most prominent on the side of the hand that is preferentially in the mouth (ie, right cheek if the right thumb is being sucked). Treatment requires behavioral modification, frequent use of bland emollients, and occasional use of low-potency topical steroids. Likewise, irritant diaper dermatitis is the most common form of diaper dermatitis and is attributable to exposure to skin irritants like feces, urine, and detergents or wipes used to cleanse the area. Treatment involves keeping the area as clean and dry as possible (eg, frequent diaper changes with higher absorbancy diapers), utilizing drying pastes or powders, avoiding harsh detergents and vigorous scrubbing/washing, and judiciously using low-potency topical steroids in short-pulsed courses when necessary.

Irritant hand dermatitis is also common in children; the most common source of exposure is excessive hand washing. Harsh detergent soaps break down the natural fat-rich substances in the skin's extracellular matrix. Repetitive exposure to water (without appropriate moisturization afterward) can also damage the epidermal skin barrier and result in transepidermal water loss. Cardinal clinical findings include patchy erythema, scaling, and fissuring concentrated on the dorsal hands and web spaces. Treatment includes avoidance of harsh detergents (in favor of nondetergent gentle cleansers), decrease in frequency of hand washing, aggressive moisturization with bland emollients, and short-pulse use of mid- to high-potency topical steroids cautiously with flares.

Children may also develop ICD on the feet. Causative exposures include moisture from occlusive shoes and mechanical friction. Hyperhidrosis is an important contributing factor. A particularly common eruption on the feet of children is juvenile plantar dermatosis (also known as "sweaty sock syndrome"). Clinical features include red, shiny, scaly, and fissured skin concentrated on the balls of the feet, heels, and plantar pads of the toes. Juvenile plantar dermatosis needs to be differentiated from ACD from shoe materials such as chromates, rubber chemicals, and fabric dyes. Distinguishing features include the fact that ACD on the feet typically involves the dorsum, whereas juvenile plantar dermatosis favors the pressure areas on the plantar foot surfaces. Treatment of juvenile plantar dermatosis includes keeping the feet cool and dry, avoiding occlusive footwear, changing socks frequently, and moisturizing the affected areas with bland emollients. Particularly painful or difficult fissures (cracks) can be treated with liquid bandages or superglue. Fortunately, the condition tends to be self-limited and resolves during puberty.

Allergic Contact Dermatitis

ACD is a delayed-type hypersensitivity reaction elicited by contact with a specific chemical on skin that has been previously sensitized. The classic appearance of ACD in the acute phase includes vesicular, weeping, crusted eczematous patches or plaques, with geometric well-demarcated borders corresponding to areas of direct chemical contact. Linear streaks are the hallmark of ACD due to poison ivy (Figure 24-1). In the chronic phase, ACD may be more thickened (lichenified), scaly, and/or hyperpigmented. The most common causes of ACD in children are plants in the *Toxicodendron* genus (eg, poison ivy), nickel, topical antibiotics, preservative chemicals (eg, formaldehyde releasing preservatives), rubber accelerators, *p*-tert-butylformaldehyde resin (associated with sports gear and sports shoes), and fragrances. Less common emerging agents include para-phenylenediamine (black hair dye) in *black henna* tattoos, cocamidopropyl betaine (CAPB) (a nonionic surfactant in "no tears" shampoos and cleansers), and disperse dyes in clothing materials.

Diagnosis of ACD relies on a having a high index of suspicion, careful investigation of exposures, and if indicated epicutaneous patch testing by a dermatologist. Patch testing,

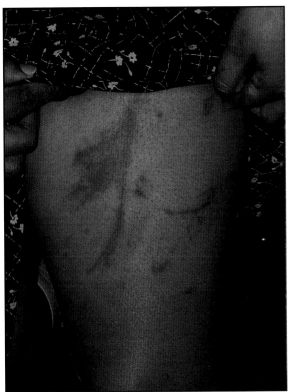

Figure 24-1. ACD from *Toxicodendron* genus plants (eg, poison ivy). Linear streaks are characteristic and correspond to areas of direct contact with the plant's oleoresin.

which detects delayed-type hypersensitivity reactions (type-IV reactions), differs from prick testing, which detects immediate-type hypersensitivity reactions.

Pruritus tends to be the dominant symptom in ACD, whereas burning and discomfort may be more common in ICD. However, differentiating ICD from ACD by clinical examination alone is often difficult, especially in chronic forms.

Generally, the location of the eruption approximates the site of greatest allergen exposure. For example, nickel dermatitis may present on the earlobes from nickel-containing earrings or in the infraumbilical area due to nickel-containing belt buckles or snaps on blue jeans ("jean snap dermatitis"). At times, however, a suspect allergen does not coincide exactly with the expected location, in what is termed *ectopic ACD*. These ectopic reactions are common in the case of allergy to tosylamide/formaldehyde in nail polish, in which case the eruption typically involves the thin skin of the eyelids or neck and spares the relatively thicker and more-protected skin of the hands and fingers. Additionally, distant and/or widespread eruptions (commonly referred to as "Id" reactions) can often be triggered by localized ACD to such chemicals as nickel and poison ivy.

NICKEL

The classic picture of nickel dermatitis is an eruption on the earlobes or periumbilical area (Figure 24-2) resulting from contact with costume jewelry (earrings), jean snaps, zippers, and/or buttons. That being said, as many as 50% of children with nickel-induced ACD can present with more diffuse reactions (known as "Id" reactions) whereby pruritic papules emerge in nonexposed sites such as on the extremities and upper trunk.

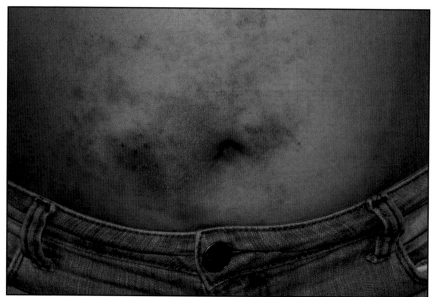

Figure 24-2. ACD due to nickel. This periumbilical distribution is a classic presentation of so-called "jean snap dermatitis."

The mainstay of treatment is avoidance of any exposure to costume jewelry, metal buckles, and snaps found in clothing such as blue jeans. Confirmatory testing for nickel offers a definitive means to discriminate clothing and personal items containing nickel. Fortunately, an easy-to-use nickel test kit is commercially available. The test involves adding a drop of 1% dimethylglyoxime-ammonia to a cotton tip applicator and rubbing the applicator against the metal in question. (Available from Dormer Laboratories Inc, Rexdale, Ontario, www.dormer.com and www.allergeaze.com.) The applicator will turn pink if the object contains nickel at a concentration of at least 1:10,000.

TOPICAL ANTIBIOTICS

Neomycin, gentamicin, and bacitracin are topical antibiotics with high rates of allergic contact sensitization in children. Additionally, cases of anaphylaxis caused by bacitracin have been reported, some of which were precipitated by the topical application of bacitracin to skin abrasions. Consequently, many dermatologists recommend against the use of neomycin- and bacitracin-containing topical antibiotic preparations, especially on clean surgical wounds.

FRAGRANCES

Fragrance allergy is common in the pediatric population, especially among adolescent females and children under 3 years of age. Exposure is usually due to the use of personal care products and perfumes or aromatic chemicals found in topical products such as make up, moisturizers, or deodorants. Typical sites of involvement include areas of greatest contact, such as the face, neck, and axilla. It is important to note that "unscented" and "scent-free" products may contain masking fragrances. Consequently, fragrance-sensitive individuals must scrutinize ingredient labels thoroughly to make sure they are truly "fragrance free."

PRESERVATIVES AND VEHICLES

ACD in children is increasingly being attributed to preservative and vehicle chemicals. One top allergen, lanolin (aka wool wax alcohols) is derived from sheep sebum, and it is used in topical medicaments and moisturizers for its emulsifying and hydrating properties. Quaternium 15, a formaldehyde releasing preservative, has been found to be among the top six allergens. Notably 3.6% of patients under the age of 18 had clinically relevant reactions.

Methylchloroisothiazolinone/methylisothiazolinone (also known as Kathon CG, and Euxyl K100) is also somewhat ubiquitous preservative chemical found to be prevalent in this population; it is used in infant products such as baby wipes, protective creams, and liquid soaps and shampoos. Heightened suspicion should be maintained for allergy to preservative and vehicle chemicals in patients who are frequently exposed to topical agents (such as children with atopic dermatitis).

TOPICAL STEROIDS

The very same topical products used to treat eczematous eruptions can at times result in allergic sensitization. A typical scenario illustrating topical steroid allergy is a child with atopic dermatitis that flares despite aggressive topical therapy. The allergy may be due to the corticosteroid itself or to an inactive ingredient (eg, preservative chemical) in the product. Patch testing to topical corticosteroids should be considered in atopic patients who appear to have exacerbations after topical steroid use or who fail to improve.

ADDITIONAL ALLERGENS

Thiuram is a compound used in rubber production and can be found in gloves and shoes. Alternative exposures in children can include pacifiers, toys, and sporting gear. In addition to thiuram, *p*-tert-butylphenol formaldehyde (an adhesive chemical) and potassium dichromate (found in tanned leather) are other allergens often present in shoe materials (Figure 24-3). Para-phenylenediamine is a common hair-dye chemical that has recently been used to enhance the color of henna tattoos (aka black henna). An increased prevalence of this allergen has been noted in the pediatric population. Disperse dyes in textiles may also be important allergens in this population, especially from school uniforms. Disperse dyes have also been associated with ACD from diaper materials. CAPB is a quaternary ammonium detergent that is found in many "no tears" shampoos. Recent evidence suggests that CAPB may be an important allergen in pediatric patients.

TREATMENT

The cornerstone of treatment of ACD is proper avoidance of the causative chemical. Topical and oral steroids play an adjunctive role, and their use should ideally be restricted to short-term symptomatic use. In cases of widespread and severe reactions, such as from poison ivy exposure, we recommend at least 3 weeks of oral prednisone with a taper in combination with topical therapy. Shorter courses often lead to rebound flares of the dermatitis. Weeping or vesicular lesions can be treated with moist cool compresses. Mild cases of dermatitis may be treated with low- to mid-potency topical steroids for several weeks. As with any topical steroid, the risk of atrophy, telangiectasias, tachyphylaxis, and

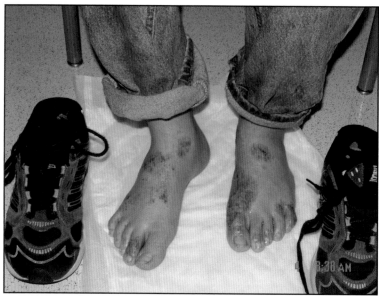

Figure 24-3. ACD to shoe materials. Well-demarcated, somewhat geometric eczematous lesions on the dorsal feet in a distribution corresponding to the patient's sneaker liner are compelling for an allergic etiology to this eruption.

systemic absorption should be kept in mind, especially in areas of increased sensitivity such as the face, groin, and flexural areas.

Once an allergen is identified, patients must be adequately educated on potential exposures and preventive measures. A recent milestone in the treatment of ACD was the creation of the Contact Allergen Management Program by the American Contact Dermatitis Society. Members of this organization are able to create customized allergen-free personal product lists for patients. (Available at www.contactderm.org.)

Summary

ICD and ACD are quite common in the pediatric population. The diagnosis rests on having a high index of suspicion, conducting a careful exposure history, and recognizing the cardinal clinical features. Treatment involves appropriate avoidance of causative exposures and implementing an appropriate treatment regimen.

Suggested Readings

Jacob SE, Brod BA, Crawford GH. Clinically relevant patch test reactions in children—a United States based study. *Pediatr Dermatol.* 2008;25(5):520-527.

Jacob SE, Burk CJ, Connelly EA. Patch testing: another steroid-spearing agent to consider in children. *Pediatr Dermatol.* 2008;25(1):81-87.

Lee PW, Elsaie ML, Jacob SE. Allergic contact dermatitis in children: common allergens and treatment: a review. *Curr Opin Pediatr.* 2009;21(4):491-498.

Militello G, Jacob SE, Crawford GH. Allergic contact dermatitis in children. *Curr Opin Pediatr.* 2006;18(4):385-390.

Zug KA, McGinley-Smith D, Warshaw EM, et al. Contact allergy in children referred for patch testing: North American Contact Dermatitis Group Data, 2001-2004. *Arch Dermatol.* 2008;144(10):1329-1336.

SECTION IV

ATOPIC DERMATITIS

What Is the Natural Progression of Atopic Dermatitis?

Lisa Arkin, MD

Eczema is the most common inflammatory skin disease in childhood. The reported prevalence in industrialized countries is between 15% and 20%, which represents a significant increase over the last 20 years. The disease course can be extremely variable. Many children have mild disease requiring intermittent use of topical medications, while others are severe and refractory necessitating chronic treatment with topical medications, light therapy, or systemic immunosuppressives. Atopic dermatitis typically starts at age 2 to 3 months and is often most exuberant on the bilateral cheeks, extensor arms and legs. If atopic dermatitis is most prominent on the bilateral cheeks in a toddler, it may be due to chronic irritant dermatitis from saliva (drooling; Figure 25-1). This, often exuberant, dermatitis can be especially recalcitrant if a child is thumb sucking or putting their hands in their mouth and then trapping saliva against the skin (see Figure 25-1). Baby wipes also can cause irritant dermatitis when used on the cheeks. Atopic dermatitis will then often generalize but becomes more prominent on the antecubital and popliteal fossae, posterior neck, ankles, and wrists in older children. Some children grow out of the condition by late childhood while others suffer from a more protracted course that relapses and remits into adulthood. Finally, some children progress to develop the "atopic march" of allergic disease, including rhinitis, allergies, and asthma, while others show no increased risk of developing asthma or allergies. This has led some to suggest the existence of 2 distinct forms of eczema, only one of which is mediated by the allergic response and should be referred to as atopic dermatitis. The diversity inherent in the disease itself makes it impossible to definitively predict prognosis for any given child at the time of diagnosis.

In recent years, however, a number of studies have helped to better define the spectrum of severity and natural progression of eczema. Some of these studies have been limited by small sample size, short duration of follow-up, and referral bias, as most patients were recruited from large academic centers more likely to follow patients with severe or refractory disease. The most positive prognostic outlook was suggested in a study by Vickers et al, which found a 90% clearance rate among 2,000 children who were

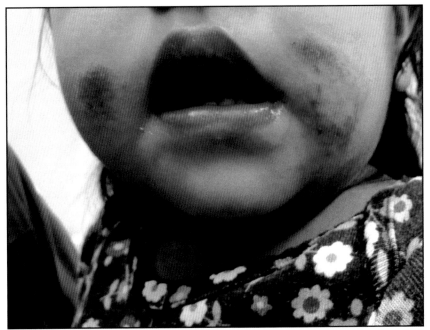

Figure 25-1. Exuberant dermatitis on bilateral cheeks. Saliva is trapped against the skin when the child's hand is in her mouth, leading to an irritant dermatitis.

followed over 10 years. A study of 870 British children by Williams and Strachan found that nearly 66% were diagnosed with eczema by the age of 7 years, suggesting an early onset of disease, and that 66% of all children were entirely clear by age 16 years. Among those who did not clear entirely, they found that a significant proportion went on to experience mild disease with intermittent relapses. Other studies, however, have suggested a less rosy prognosis with clearance rates of 30% to 70% by late adolescence.

In addition, numerous investigations have attempted to clarify the relationship between eczema and the development of the "atopic march," which includes asthma, allergies, and allergic rhinitis. Some of these studies, detailed next, should be interpreted with caution as they utilized either skin-prick testing or radioallergosorbent tests (RAST, which measure antigen-specific immunoglobulin E levels) to quantify allergic disease in study patients. The specificity of these tests is low (approximately 30% to 50%), which means that each result must be interpreted in the context of a patient's clinical reaction. Many patients will have positive test results without ever having had a clinical reaction.

Illi et al studied 1314 children from birth to age 7 years and found a cumulative eczema prevalence of approximately 20% in the first 2 years of life. The strongest risk factors for poor prognosis were the severity of disease at presentation, elevated RAST, and a parental history of eczema. No other variables—including sex, breast-feeding, pet keeping, cat allergen exposure, parental smoking, number of older siblings, and recurrence of infectious diseases—were associated with the manifestation or phenotypic severity eczema. Children with early onset eczema (before the age of 2 years) were more likely to develop asthma than those with later-onset disease. However, the majority of children with early-onset eczema who *also* developed asthma had experienced episodes of wheezing before the age of 3 years. Those with eczema in the absence of early-onset wheezing showed no increased risk for developing asthma than other children. Among all children, approximately 40% were in complete remission by age 3 years, 40% demonstrated an intermittent pattern of disease, and 20% had yearly symptoms through the age of 7 years.

Further, Kussel et al prospectively studied a birth cohort of 263 children who were followed for eczema and allergies over 5 years. Among all subjects, 66% developed eczema within the first 5 years; 85% of these reported a rash within the first year. Two-thirds of patients had positive skin-prick testing. The patients with positive skin-prick testing, who were deemed "atopic," were more likely to be male, to have persistent eczema at 5 years, and to have been diagnosed with asthma or allergic rhinitis. The remaining one of three "nonatopic" eczema patients, whose skin-prick tests remained negative at 5 years, were more likely to be female and present with eczema later in childhood, and they were less likely to carry the diagnosis of asthma or allergic rhinitis at 5 years. Finally, Novembre et al followed a group of 111 children between the ages of 2 and 11 and found no increased risk of asthma in children with eczema whose skin-prick tests were negative to common food and inhalant allergens. Collectively, this evidence suggests that not all eczema is mediated by allergy and atopic dermatitis should therefore, be thought of as a separate entity. The "nonatopic" variant of eczema may be driven by an entirely distinct mechanism that is currently unknown.

In addition, a subpopulation of patients with eczema have mutations in the filaggrin gene, which encodes a protein that plays a key role in the barrier formation of the stratum corneum. Filaggrin mutations appear to be one of the strongest genetic risk factors for developing severe atopic disease, as decreased or absent expression leads to impaired barrier function, allowing for the entry of environmental antigens and allergens. Multiple studies have confirmed that eczema patients with loss-of-function mutations in filaggrin develop early-onset, persistent disease along with asthma and atopic sensitization. However, routine screening for this mutation is not currently utilized in clinical practice. It is not currently known whether early intervention in children with filaggrin mutations might alter the trajectory of this disease and the risk for secondary atopic outcomes.

Summary

Eczema is an inflammatory disease with a wide spectrum of disease activity. Patients with filaggrin mutations share a genetic basis for the disease but little is definitively known about other predisposing inherited or environmental factors. Patients with early-onset eczema (before the age of 2 years), severe disease at presentation, a parental history of eczema, and positive RAST to common environmental antigens are more likely to have severe and persistent eczema. Further, those with eczema and episodes of wheezing before the age of 3 years appear more likely to develop asthma than those without early-onset wheezing. In spite of this, many patients—upward of two-thirds of patients from the studies reviewed—will outgrow their eczema or develop mild disease by adolescence. Finally, patients with filaggrin mutations are more likely to have more severe persistent disease associated with allergies and asthma, but it is not known whether early intervention for these patients will alter the course of their disease.

Suggested Readings

Henderson J, Northstone K, Lee S, et al. The burden of disease associated with filaggrin mutations: a population-based, longitudinal birth cohort study. *J Allergy Clin Immunol*. 2008;121(4):872-877.

Illi S, von Mutius E, Lau S, Nickel R, Gruber C, Niggemann B, Wahn U; Multicenter Allergy Study Group. The natural course of atopic dermatitis from birth to age 7 years and the association with asthma. *J Allergy Clin Immunol*. 2004;113(5):925-931.

Irvine AD. Fleshing out filaggrin phenotypes. *J Invest Dermatol*. 2007;127(3):504-507.

Ker J, Hartert TV. The atopic march: what's the evidence? *Ann Allergy Asthma Immunol*. 2009;103(4):282-289.

Kusel MM, Holt PG, de Klerk N, Sly PD. Support for 2 variants of eczema. *J Allergy Clin Immunol*. 2005;116(5): 1067-1072.

Novembre E, Cianferoni A, Lombardi E, Bernardini R, Pucci N, Vierucci A. Natural history of "instrinsic" atopic dermatitis. *Allergy*. 2001;56(5):452-453.

Vickers HR. The problem of the pathogenesis of endogenous eczema. *Br J Dermatol*. 1952;65(6):225-230.

Williams HC, Strachan DP. The natural history of childhood eczema: observations from the British 1958 birth cohort study. *Br J Dermatol*. 1998;139(5):834-839.

What Are the Different Treatment Options for Atopic Dermatitis Based on Age and Affected Body Part?

James R. Treat, MD

Atopic skin care is the backbone of successful therapy for atopic dermatitis. Bathing with gentle nonsoap cleansers, frequent use of thick emollients, and avoidance of harsh fabrics and fragrances may be enough to treat mild atopic dermatitis. When this is not enough, therapy with anti-inflammatory medications is often needed. Topical steroids have a long and safe track record of use in children as long as the strength, vehicle, amount of body surface covered, and number of refills are chosen with care. Topical steroids are often used off label and this question is based on clinical experience but many of the recommendations are off-label use of FDA-approved medications. See Question 27 for a full discussion of alternatives to topical steroids for atopic dermatitis.

Therapy in atopic dermatitis should involve both maintenance and flare plans (similar to asthma care plans). Some children can be maintained for long periods with just good atopic skin care as detailed above but some may also need low-potency topical steroids or calcineurin inhibitors on a more consistent basis in order to prevent flares. Even low potency medications should not be given continuously but instead tapered to the lowest effective dose. Breaks from therapy will help avoid possible side effects. Stronger topical steroids can then be reserved for flares thus making their use safer, and likely more effective, as the skin does not get habituated to them.

It is vital to understand the side effects of the medications being used. Symptomatic adrenal insufficiency and striae are uncommon when topical steroids are used appropriately. Striae are actually more common in growing preadolescent and adolescent children than in infants and young children. Cataracts and glaucoma can occur from topical steroids and their use should be limited on the face, especially around the eyes.

All children with atopic dermatitis should be advised on good atopic skin care. Good dermatologic care is NOT just about picking the correct topical steroid. The following should be reviewed with all atopic dermatitis patients, no matter their severity.

Atopic Skin Care

- Most children will do better with infrequent bathing (every other day) for 5 to 10 minutes in lukewarm water. Children with prominent environmental allergies to cats, dogs, pollen, ragweed, dust mites, etc may do better with daily short baths to wash off allergens (see Question 29).
- Do not use washcloths/loofah/sponges. They are rough on the skin and can easily spread bacterial or viral infection if present.
- Use nonsoap cleansers or gentle cleansers (examples include Dove fragrance-free soap [Unilever, Rotterdam, Netherlands], Cetaphil gentle skin cleanser [Galderma Laboratories, Ft. Worth, TX], or Vanicream cleansing bar [Pharmaceutical Specialties, Inc, Rochester, MN]).
- Moisturize with thick emollients that are creams or ointments and apply them twice daily. Emollients are particularly effective when the skin is wet after bathing. Typically, if an emollient is a cream or ointment, it will come in a jar or tube and will be very thick and much less likely to burn the open skin of children with atopic dermatitis. Lotions (which generally come out of pump bottles) are generally NOT as effective as moisturizers and many patients will complain they burn and thus refuse use.
- When prescribing, whenever possible, use topical steroids ointments. Cream formulations of medication often burn, leading to children refusing therapy. Note that ointment versions of the same medication and percentage may be stronger than their cream counterparts.
- Avoid nylon and wool-containing clothing and keep the skin covered whenever possible with soft cotton. Children with atopic dermatitis will often start itching vigorously whenever the skin is exposed or irritated and can thus precipitate a flare.

Maintenance Therapy General Guidelines

MILD-TO-MODERATE ATOPIC DERMATITIS

- Consistent moisturization and good atopic skin care are often adequate for mild-to-moderate atopic dermatitis (Figures 26-1 and 26-2).
- Another option is a premixed amount of a low potency topical steroid in a moisturizer. A common formula is 5 g of hydrocortisone Acetate powder in 454 g of moisturizer (such as petrolatum) giving a 1.25% hydrocortisone mixture by weight. This can be used alternately with a plain moisturizer and then tapered to every other day or less or increased to twice daily depending on need. Alternatively, if the insurance does not cover a premixed formulation, it is simple for parents to mix 2.5% hydrocortisone in the hand with a plain moisturizer in a 1:1 concentration and end up with the same 1.25% hydrocortisone mixture. This also allows the parents to titrate the amount of steroid to what is needed. For instance, on days when the skin is clear, the plain

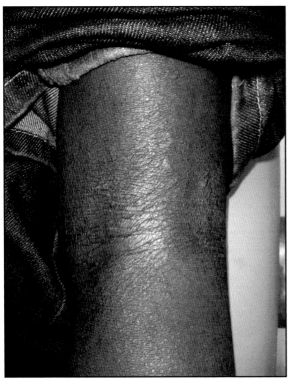

Figure 26-1. Dry scaling patches on the popliteal fossae with follicular accentuation.

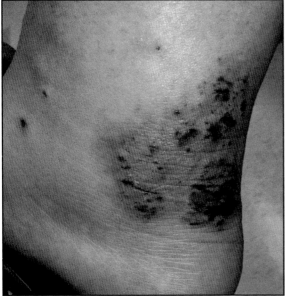

Figure 26-2. Localized lichenified and excoriated plaque of atopic dermatitis on the ankle.

moisturizer is used and with very early flares the topical steroid can be mixed back in by hand to a greater or lesser extent depending on need. The steroid can be mixed in more in circumstances such as season changes when flares are more likely. Even this low-potency topical steroid does need to be monitored and its use restricted to limited amounts of time especially in young children and skin folds.

SEVERE ATOPIC DERMATITIS

- Good atopic skin care.
- Premixed amount of a low-potency topical steroid in the moisturizer as denoted previously such as 5 g of hydrocortisone powder in 454 g of moisturizer giving a 1.25% hydrocortisone mix by weight can be used as detailed before.
- Low- to mid-potency topical steroids may also be used 2 to 3 times weekly with just moisturizer on the days when the medication is not used. This therapy has been tested in children (older than 1 year of age) but should be monitored very carefully and limited to the shortest amount of time and medication necessary.

Flare Guidelines

Most topical steroids and calcineurin inhibitors are not approved for use in infants and young children but atopic dermatitis must be treated in this age group to make children comfortable, prevent infection, and help to maintain healthy growth and development not hindered by constant itching and poor sleeping. For flares, appropriate-strength topical steroids (as outlined below) can often be used safely for 2 to 3 weeks at a time but should always be tapered as soon as possible. Pimecrolimus is indicated in children over 2 years, tacrolimus 0.03% is indicated in children 2 to 15 years, and tacrolimus 0.1% over 15 years old, and these can serve as steroid-sparing agents. There is a black box warning on calcineurin inhibitors for the risk of cancer.

For discussion of other therapeutic measures, please see Questions 27 and 29.

Bottom Line

There is a general fear of topical steroids and calcineurin inhibitors among patients and providers. I have tried to outline guidelines for safe and effective use of topical steroids, but some of this information is off label based on experience and it must always be tailored to individual patients. You will often find that if you use appropriately strong topical steroids for a short period of time, and then give families reasonable maintenance plans along with counseling on good atopic skin care, you will use less total medication.

LOCATION-SPECIFIC THERAPY FOR FLARES

- Face, neck, axillae, inguinal folds, buttocks folds, and other major skin folds (under breasts in teenage women) are the most sensitive skin, may absorb topical steroids more easily, and be more susceptible to skin thinning and striae. Therefore, topical steroids should be used very minimally here.

○ For flares: Class-VII topical steroids for 1 to 2 weeks and in older children class-VI steroids for 1 to 2 weeks.

- Trunk and arms and legs can often tolerate low- to mid-potency steroids (if over 1 year) for 1 to 2 weeks for flares but be aware the antecubital and popliteal fossae are also major skin folds so these areas need to be monitored, and the use of topical steroids should not be continued for extended times.
- Hands, feet, elbows, and knees have the thickest skin and can tolerate and often need stronger topical steroids.

AGE-SPECIFIC THERAPY

Children ages 3 to 12 months should not have consistent topical steroids used and generally low-potency topical steroids are used for short periods of time for flares and then atopic skin-care is used for maintenance. If children at this age cannot be weaned off of topical steroids in between flares they should be referred to a specialist for management. There are some topical steroids approved for use in this age group but again for limited times. For instance, alclometasone ointment 0.05% is approved for use over 1 year of age. Ultrapotent topical steroids, such as clobetasol propionate 0.05%, are generally not indicated for children with atopic dermatitis.

Suggested Readings

Friedlander SF, Hebert A, Allen DB. Safety of fluticasone propionate cream 0.05% for the treatment of severe and extensive atopic dermatitis in children as young as 3 months. *J Am Acad Dermatol.* 2002;46(3):387-393.

Hong E, Smith S, Fischer G. Evaluation of the atrophogenic potential of topical corticosteroids in pediatric dermatology patients. *Pediatr Dermatol.* 2011;28(4):393-396. doi:10.1111/j.1525-1470.2011.01445.x. Epub 2011 Apr 20.

Thomas KS, Armstrong S, Avery A, et al. Randomised controlled trial of short bursts of a potent topical corticosteroid versus prolonged use of a mild preparation for children with mild or moderate atopic eczema. *BMJ.* 2002;324(7340):768-771.

What Are the Alternatives to Topical Steroids for Atopic Dermatitis?

Marissa J. Perman, MD

Background

Atopic dermatitis (AD) is a multifactorial T-cell-mediated disease characterized by recurrent and often chronic pruritic, scaly, erythematous patches and plaques in a characteristic distribution depending on the age of the patient. While topical steroids are the mainstay of treatment for this common condition, alternative topical therapies may also improve symptoms. Topical steroids are safe when used appropriately, but substitute therapies are often required due to the risk of side effects associated with frequent and inappropriate steroid use. These side effects include atrophy, dyspigmentation, tachyphylaxis, telangiectasias, systemic absorption with possible risk for hypothalamic-pituitary axis dysfunction, and steroid addiction.

Alternative therapies should be considered in patients requiring frequent or long-term management of their disease. Topical treatment alternatives that I commonly use include emollients, barrier-repair lipid moisturizers, and topical calcineurin inhibitors (TCIs; Table 27-1). Oral antihistamines also have a role, albeit limited, in controlling pruritus associated with AD. Due to the susceptibility of bacterial infections in patients with AD, antibiotics play a role. Finally, systemic immunosuppressive agents and phototherapy will briefly be discussed.

Emollients

Severe dryness (xerosis) is highly associated with AD, and therefore, emollients have an important role in AD management. In patients with AD, the normal skin barrier is disrupted, leading to transepidermal water loss, exposure to allergens, and susceptibility to several infectious agents including *Staphylococcus aureus (S aureus)* and herpes simplex virus. Therefore, repair of the abnormal barrier and prevention of transepidermal water

---

Table 27-1

Alternatives to Topical Steroid Therapy Based on Atopic Dermatitis Severity

Atopic Dermatitis Severity	Alternatives to Topical Steroid Therapy
Mild	• Emollients • Emollients + barrier-repair lipid moisturizers
Moderate	• Emollients + barrier-repair lipid moisturizers • Emollients + TCIs
Severe	• Emollients + barrier-repair lipid moisturizers alternating with TCIs • Consider referral to dermatology

TCI indicates topical calcineurin inhibitor

---

loss with emollients is critical. Emollients are safe in large quantities, and I encourage application multiple times a day.

Families are often overwhelmed by the wide selection of available lotions, creams, and ointments. Ointments tend to be more occlusive than creams and lotions and help to better retain moisture in the skin. You can tell your patients that thicker emollients (creams and ointments) are more beneficial for xerosis than lotions. Generally, if emollients come in a tub, then they are thick creams or ointments. If they come in a pump bottle, they are less occlusive and may burn when applied to open skin. However, these characteristics must be balanced with the patient's and family's personal preferences. Some patients are very resistant to using a thick, greasy ointment, such as petrolatum, and would be better off with a cream as long as it is applied consistently. In addition, patients may tolerate a thicker emollient at night than during the day. Emollients should be applied immediately (within 3 minutes) after bathing when the patient's skin is still slightly moist, which helps to seal in the moisture. Ideally, emollients should be applied at least twice a day, and dye-free, fragrance-free products are best suited for patients with AD.

Over the past several years, new nonsteroidal barrier-repair lipid moisturizers have become available and provide yet another alternative to topical steroids. The outermost layer of the epidermis, known as the stratum corneum, forms a lipid-laden barrier to retain moisture in the skin. The most prevalent lipids in the stratum corneum are ceramides, with cholesterol and free fatty acids comprising the rest. Several moisturizers containing variable proportions of these lipids are available including Epiceram and CeraVe. CeraVe does not require a prescription.

Two other nonsteroidal prescription barrier-repair therapies that have shown to be useful in some patients include Atopiclair and Mimyx. Atopiclair is a barrier-repair and anti-inflammatory cream containing glycyrrhetinic acid, hyaluronic acid, and lipids. Mimyx contains palmitoylethanolamide, an endogenous bioactive fatty acid and an important component of the skin barrier that is deficient in atopic skin. Both medications require a prescription, and the cost may be prohibitive for some patients.

Barrier-repair moisturizers are advertised to improve AD and alleviate pruritus, pain, and burning. Patients with mild-to-moderate AD may be able to use these topical preparations as maintenance therapies. Those with more severe disease will likely still require topical steroids and/or TCIs for flares but can use barrier-repair lipid moisturizers for milder disease.

Other Topical Immunomodulators

My next step on the potency ladder of topical therapeutic agents is TCIs. TCIs should be considered in patients who do not respond to the above therapies. I use TCIs in a similar fashion to topical steroids (ie, once or twice daily to the affected areas during disease flares followed by discontinuation when clear). They can also be alternated with topical steroids every 2 weeks to minimize the side effects from steroids. TCIs are useful for thinner skin such as the face and genitals where side effects due to steroids are more likely to occur despite limited use. They include tacrolimus Protopic ointment 0.03% and Elidel cream 1%. TCIs block cytokine production by activated T-cells and mast cells, reducing inflammation in AD. They are FDA approved as a second-line therapy for moderate-to-severe AD in children age 2 years and older. Protopic ointment 0.1% is approved for patients age 16 years and older.

TCIs are well tolerated with minimal side effects and are safe to use for extended periods of time. Occasionally, patients complain of a burning or stinging sensation following application especially when applied to broken-down skin. Families should be counseled about the black box warning regarding carcinogenic potential. Although the FDA states that no causal link has been found, the black box warning stems from a theoretical risk of malignancy found in animal studies and safety profiles and reported malignancies in patients taking oral calcineurin inhibitors. Postmarketing surveillance studies are under way, but most prescribing physicians believe TCIs are safe and have minimal, if any, systemic absorption in most patients.

Other Approaches

The role of probiotics in the management of AD is still under investigation. Results of studies evaluating both maternal and infant supplementation of probiotics have found conflicting results. Similar conflicting results have been found in the role of breast feeding and the introduction of solid foods as they relate to the development or prevention of AD. Further long-term studies are needed before definitive recommendations can be made.

Systemic Medications

Oral antihistamines play a limited but important role in AD-associated pruritus, the etiology of which is not entirely clear. Most studies do not support the role of histamine in AD, and therefore, oral antihistamines should not have a primary role in management. However, I recommend first-generation antihistamines for their sedative properties particularly at night when pruritus is often more severe.

Antibiotics, while not a direct alternative to topical steroids, play a significant role in decreasing erythema, crust, and oozing associated with secondary infections commonly seen in patients with chronic AD. Bacterial colonization and growth, most notably *S aureus,* is frequently encountered in AD and should be considered as a possible etiology to a sudden flare. I recommend obtaining a culture prior to treating to evaluate for evidence of methicillin-resistant *S aureus* or other resistance and adjusting the antimicrobials accordingly. In addition, diluted sodium hypochlorite (bleach) baths help to decrease colonization (refer to Reference 4, Hanifin et al, for preparing a bleach bath).

Finally, I will briefly comment about systemic therapy as an alternative to topical steroids. AD is a T-cell-mediated disease that is responsive to systemic immunomodulating agents. Oral corticosteroids will dramatically improve AD in most cases; however, patients tend to flare upon discontinuation. The flare may be more severe than the patient's baseline skin disease and can lead to a vicious cycle with patients often requesting oral corticosteroid therapy as a quick fix. Thus, oral steroids should generally be avoided in treating AD.

There are several steroid-sparing agents that can be used in the management of chronic, recalcitrant AD unresponsive to topical therapy, including cyclosporine, azathioprine, and mycophenolate mofetil. Cyclosporine is probably the most frequently used agent in children and can be used as short-term monotherapy before returning to topical therapies or as a bridge to other steroid-sparing agents. Both low-dose (2.5 mg/kg/day) and high-dose (5 mg/kg/day) cyclosporine intermittently or continuously for up to 1 year have been used with success in children.

Cyclosporine, azathioprine, and mycophenolate mofetil have multiple side effects and require frequent laboratory monitoring. Most of these medications do not provide long-term remission, and the disease often flares upon discontinuation. Cyclosporine, however, has been shown to improve the overall extent of disease after discontinuation.

Narrowband ultraviolet B phototherapy is another systemic option in more severe cases of pediatric AD, which may provide significant benefit for several months after discontinuation. Phototherapy can down regulate the immune response by reducing DNA synthesis and may be a good option for children in need of systemic treatment without the adverse effects associated with other oral systemic medications. However, it requires multiple treatments each week that can be challenging in school-aged children. Other risks associated with phototherapy are related to frequent sun exposure such as erythema, photoaging, and the theoretical risk of skin cancer.

Patients should be referred to a dermatologist for further evaluation and management when the above-mentioned therapies are not effective. Severe and recalcitrant AD may require systemic therapy and consideration for alternative diagnoses.

Suggested Readings

Amor KT, Ryan C, Menter A. The use of cyclosporine in dermatology: part I. *J Am Acad Dermatol.* 2010;63(6):925-946; quiz 947-8.

Carbone A, Siu A, Patel R. Pediatric atopic dermatitis: a review of the medical management. *Ann Pharmacother.* 2010;44(9):1448-1458.

Chamlin SL, Kao J, Frieden IJ, et al. Ceramide-dominant barrier repair lipids alleviate childhood atopic dermatitis: changes in barrier function provide a sensitive indicator of disease activity. *J Am Acad Dermatol.* 2002;47(2): 198-208.

Hanifin JM, Paller AS, Eichenfield L, et al. US Tacrolimus Ointment Study Group. Efficacy and safety of tacrolimus ointment treatment for up to 4 years in patients with atopic dermatitis. *J Am Acad Dermatol.* 2005;53(2 Suppl 2): S186-S194.

Krakowski AC, Eichenfield LF, Dohil MA. Management of atopic dermatitis in the pediatric population. *Pediatrics.* 2008;122(4):812-824.

HOW DO I DIAGNOSE AND MANAGE ECZEMA HERPETICUM?

Andrea L. Zaenglein, MD

While eczema herpeticum, also known as Kaposi varioliform eruption, is not a common complication of atopic dermatitis, it is a classic example of how a defective skin barrier can allow for widespread, exaggerated infection. Herpes simplex virus (HSV) with primary or recurrent infection can disseminate over eczematous skin instead of remaining localized as is typically seen. Persons with other skin diseases that damage the epidermal barrier, such as Darier disease, Hailey-Hailey disease, bullous pemphigus, pemphigus foliaceus, ichthyosis vulgaris, and burns, can also experience eczema herpeticum. Defects in the innate immunity, evidenced by low cathelicidin and β-defensin levels, and specific defects in the gene encoding filaggrin, an important structural protein in the skin, explain why the virus is not held in check by the body's immune system. Clinically, risk factors for eczema herpeticum include head and neck involvement of atopic dermatitis and having more severe and generalized disease. While HSV1 is more common, HSV2 can also cause eczema herpeticum. Children with atopic dermatitis have altered skin immunity with lowered innate immunity thus leading to an increased risk of infection. Children who have a history of eczema herpeticum are even more likely to experience secondary bacterial infections and infection with molluscum.

Diagnosing eczema herpeticum can be difficult especially early on in the course when it can be misdiagnosed as impetigo or folliculitis. It is important to think of eczema herpeticum whenever there is pain or fever associated with a flare of eczema. Typically, hemorrhagic-crusted vesicles or punched out erosions are disseminated over the face, neck, and upper trunk (Figure 28-1). Children often feel and look quite miserable. Secondary infections with *Staphylococcus aureus (S aureus)* can also occur, further complicating the picture and leading to significant morbidity and mortality if untreated. The differential diagnosis includes eczema vaccinatum, a disseminated smallpox infection seen in patients with atopic dermatitis exposed to a person recently vaccinated against smallpox. Currently only military personnel are being immunized against smallpox. Also, Coxsackie A16 (hand, foot, and mouth disease) and primary bacterial superinfection of eczema should be considered.

Figure 28-1. A 12-year-old boy with severe, generalized atopic dermatitis presenting with fever, malaise, and wide spread vesicles on face and neck.

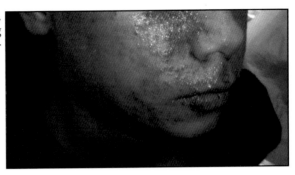

Direct fluorescence antibody testing is a widely available and rapid test for HSV. Results are available in just a couple of hours. If negative, a polymerase chain reaction (PCR) (if available) or viral culture can be done. Viral culture is specific but not always sensitive, whereas, PCR is the most sensitive and specific option but not widely available. Tzanck smear, a direct look at infected cells on a microscope slide, can also rapidly confirm a diagnosis of HSV but is limited by the need for stain, microscope, and an experienced microscopist. In older lesions, a skin biopsy is best at detecting herpesvirus infection. This is usually done in atypical or chronic HSV infections. Antibody titers to HSV may not detect early infection and have a high-false positive rate for immunoglobulin M (IgM). Testing should be done with these limits in mind (Table 28-1).

Once the diagnosis of eczema herpeticum is confirmed, or even if there is high clinical suspicion for infection, treatment should be initiated. Antivirals, which work by inhibiting viral replication, are most effective when given early in the course so treatment should not be delayed. It is important to consider the physical state of the child when deciding whether to treat as an outpatient or to admit to the hospital. There is no clear consensus on acyclovir dosing for eczema herpeticum. In otherwise healthy, older children who have no comorbid factors, are stable, and not dehydrated, oral acyclovir can be given. Mucocutaneous dosing of acyclovir is typically used (children over 2 years of age: 1200 mg/day divided q8hr with max 80 mg/kg/day). Therapy is typically continued for 7 to 10 days or until fully crusted over. Close monitoring should be done to ensure adequate treatment response. Make sure to counsel the parents to continue aggressive treatment of the underlying atopic dermatitis as well with topical corticosteroids and bland emollients.

If a child is very young; unable to maintain hydration; has a particularly severe, generalized infection; or if compliance is questionable, hospitalization is warranted. Intravenous acyclovir should be initiated. If treating intravenously, some advocate mucocutaneous HSV dosing (15 mg/kg/day IV divided q8hr) but for more severe cases varicella zoster dosing can be used (30 mg/kg/day IV divided q8hr). Children with recurrent eczema herpeticum should be put on suppressive antiviral therapy to prevent additional outbreaks. Typical dosing for suppression is the same as would be given for suppression of mucocutaneous HSV. Valacyclovir is only approved for children over 2 years of age for varicella. Some advocate the use of valacyclovir as an off-label option for treatment or prophylaxis of eczema herpeticum.

Table 28-1

Testing for Herpes Simplex Virus

Test	How Performed	Pros/Cons
DFA	Scrape vesicle with surgical blade (#15). Apply cells to glass microscope slide.	• Quick (1 to 2 hours) • Inexpensive • Able to tell HSV1 from HSV2
Tzanck test	Scrape vesicle with surgical blade (#15). Apply cells to glass microscope slide. Stain with Giemsa (or Wright) stain. Examine under microscope.	• Quickest • Inexpensive • Can be highly inaccurate, depending on who processes and interprets the slide
Viral culture	Deroof vesicle with surgical blade (#15). Swab vesicle base with viral specific swab and place in viral culture medium.	• Accurate (if positive) • High false negative rate • Not quick (1 to 3 days)
PCR	Done on cells, fluid, or blood.	• Can differentiate HSV1 and HSV2 • Sensitive, but false positives and false negatives can occur
Serologic testing	Blood test for IgM, IgG antibodies to HSV.	• High rate false-positive IgM
Biopsy	A skin biopsy is taken and sent for H&E stain.	• Very accurate if positive • Good for unusual or older lesions • Cannot differentiate HSV1 and HSV2

DFA indicates direct fluorescent antibody; H&E, hematoxylin and eosin; HSV, herpes simplex virus; IgG, immunoglobulin G; IgM, immunoglobulin M; PCR, polymerase chain reaction

Secondary bacterial infections, most often with *S aureus* but also with Group A *Streptococcus*, are common in widespread cases of eczema herpeticum. It is important to perform a bacterial culture in addition to viral cultures in suspected individuals. Colonization and infection with methicillin-resistant *S aureus* is not uncommon in children with atopic dermatitis. Determining antibiotic sensitivity is important to ensure adequate antimicrobial coverage.

If lesions are involving the periocular area, ophthalmology should be urgently consulted. If there is herpes keratitis present, antiviral eye drops are given in addition to systemic antiviral treatment. If after 21 days of therapy, corneal re-epithelialization has not occurred, alternate therapy should be considered.

It is important that any provider have a high index of suspicion for eczema herpeticum in children with atopic dermatitis that experience an unusual flare associated with systemic symptoms. Timely evaluation to assess severity and appropriate viral and bacterial cultures are warranted, while prompt initiation of antiviral treatment is key to preventing widespread infection and quick resolution of symptoms.

Suggested Readings

Dekker CL, Prober CG. Pediatric uses of valacyclovir, penciclovir and famciclovir. *Pediatr Infect Dis J*. 2001;20(11): 1079-1081.

Frisch S, Siegfried EC. The clinical spectrum and therapeutic challenge of eczema herpeticum. *Pediatr Dermatol*. 2011; 28(1):46-52.

Gao PS, Rafaels NM, Hand T, et al. Filaggrin mutations that confer risk of atopic dermatitis confer greater risk for eczema herpeticum. *J Allergy Clin Immunol*. 2009;124(3):507-513, 513.e1-7.

Hata TR, Kotol P, Boguniewicz M, et al. History of eczema herpeticum is associated with the inability to induce human β-defensin (HBD)-2, HBD-3 and cathelicidin in the skin of patients with atopic dermatitis. *Br J Dermatol*. 2010;163(3):659-661.

Jen M, Chang MW. Eczema herpeticum and eczema vaccinatum in children. *Pediatr Ann*. 2010;39(10):658-664.

Wollenberg A, Zoch C, Wetzel S, Plewig G, Przybilla B. Predisposing factors and clinical features of eczema herpeticum: a retrospective analysis of 100 cases. *J Am Acad Dermatol*. 2003;49(2):198-205.

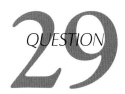

WHEN SHOULD I REFER A PATIENT WITH ECZEMA TO AN ALLERGIST?

Terri Brown-Whitehorn, MD

We know that approximately 10% to 20% of infants and children have eczema. Of those, 40% to 80% have evidence of atopy/allergy. We also know that eczema is a multifactorial disease and allergy is not the only trigger. Genetics, environmental exposures (including weather, humidity, aeroallergens, infections), diet, and underlying immune responses all play a role. So, who will benefit from an allergist's evaluation and treatment recommendations? I shall review the role of environmental allergies, food allergies, concomitant asthma, and allergic rhinitis, and although rare, underlying immunodeficiency, in patients with eczema.

We know that 85% of children with eczema present before their fifth birthday (with 60% presenting before 1 year of age). Of those, 80% have elevated total immunoglobulin E (IgE) levels and evidence of allergic sensitization.

Clues for Allergic Sensitization From the History and Examination

- Are there concomitant allergy symptoms such as itchy eyes, rhinitis, and/or nasal congestion?
- Is there a family history of environmental allergies, asthma, food allergy, or eczema?
- Does the eczema flare in certain seasons or with certain exposures?
- Is the child's eczema better at someone else's home?
- Where is the eczema located?

If the eczema is on "exposed areas" (face, hands, and feet) or if the eczema is difficult to treat, one should consider an environmental trigger. Although the role of perennial allergens in eczema is a bit controversial, my general approach is to look for perennial allergens (dust, pets, and mold) in the younger age groups and in children with year-round symptoms. I look for pollen sensitivity in children whose eczema flares in the spring or fall. Once suspected, sending specific environmental IgE testing (not panels that include food) or referring directly to an allergist is recommended. Allergy testing can sometimes lag behind clinical symptoms especially in our younger patients; however, a child does not need to be over 2 years of age to have testing. I have seen many infants and toddlers with positive testing to cats, dogs, and dust. If you think that your patient has environmental allergies, a referral to an allergist for skin-prick testing and additional education/management strategies is helpful.

There is a common misconception that all or most children with eczema have food allergies and if found, the child's eczema would be cured. Unfortunately, it is not that easy. Studies have shown that 5% of children with mild eczema, 15% to 20% of children with moderate eczema, and a third of children with severe eczema have food as a contributing factor. Only 35% to 40% of parental-reported suspicions of food allergy can be verified by oral food challenges.

Which Patients Are More Likely to Have a Food Allergy?

We need to go back to the original history and examination. In an infant or child with difficult-to-treat eczema, diffuse disease, or moderate-to-severe eczema, food allergy testing should be considered (and performed in infants). Also, by history if there is a specific food that leads to worsening of rash, then directed food allergy testing is recommended. The most common causes of food allergy in pediatrics are milk, eggs, soy, wheat, and peanuts (tree nuts, fish, and shellfish in older kids/adults). Specific IgE testing can be performed by either a primary care physician or an allergist knowledgeable in interpretation. We will check milk, eggs, soy, wheat, and peanuts (not a food panel). An allergist will use skin-prick testing to confirm food allergy. The negative predictive value of these tests is 95%. Therefore, if food allergy testing is negative, it is unlikely that the food is triggering the eczema. However, if a child has a positive test to a food, there is a 40% chance that it is a false negative test. Therefore, screening for food allergies with no indication is problematic. We do not recommend allergy testing to foods for all patients. If testing to food is positive, our typical approach is to have the child remove positive food(s) for a 4-week period. If there is no improvement, the child should resume eating the food. If there is improvement, we would recommend continued avoidance and regular follow-up with his or her allergist (may outgrow over time). In an infant or child who is breast fed or in whom testing was performed for foods that are not yet in the diet and testing was positive, there is a possibility of a severe allergic reaction with their first ingestion. I recommend and prescribe epinephrine autoinjectors to all of these children. For those with multiple food allergies, a nutrition referral is made. If the relationship between food allergy and eczema remains unclear, the gold standard is an observed oral food challenge. In summary, in an infant or child with moderate-to-severe eczema, diffuse disease, or parental concern of food allergy, directed food allergy testing can be performed and referral to an allergist is recommended. Also, patients with positive food testing should be referred to an allergist.

Patients Who Progress to Allergic Rhinitis or Asthma May Warrant a Referral to an Allergist

Whereas some children may outgrow their eczema over time, others may develop allergic rhinitis and asthma. This progression from eczema to allergic rhinitis to asthma has been studied over time and is known as the atopic march. Primary care providers need to ask about concomitant rhinitis, conjunctivitis, and cough or wheeze. Specific questions need to be asked. Although I do not feel that all children with mild asthma, allergic rhinitis, and eczema need to be seen by an allergist, I do believe that all children may benefit from an initial examination and testing. I do believe that those with more moderate-to-severe disease should see an allergist.

I also think that there is a large group of infants and children with eczema that is mild and yet primary care providers may wonder if an allergist referral would be of benefit. The decision of whether to refer may not be as easy as those with more severe disease. My typical approach in a child with mild eczema (even if it is diffuse) is thick moisturizers (cream or ointment) twice a day. Low-potency topical steroids, such as a class 6 (ie, prednicarbate) or class 7 (ie, hydrocortisone), can be applied twice a day to the affected areas (even if large area). Once improved, then I would wean to daily or even consider a few times a week (as preventative). When applying steroid cream/ointment along with moisturizers, I also recommend applying steroid medication first and then waiting 30 to 60 minutes to apply moisturizer (as to not dilute the effectiveness of the steroid). Some will also use calcineurin inhibitors for mild areas in the same manner as the lower potency steroids. However, if symptoms do not improve or if there is constant need for low-potency topical steroids or calcineurin inhibitors to be applied, OR if there is parental or provider concern, certainly an allergy referral may be helpful. I also believe that once higher potency steroids are needed on the face or if there is a persistent need for steroids on the face, we should look for a potential trigger (we often find one). I think that if there are any concerns by the family or by the primary care provider, a referral to an allergist might be helpful.

Immunodeficiency Syndromes That Can Present With Eczematous Dermatitis

Primary immunodeficiency disorders are also associated with eczema. Omenn syndrome, a form of severe combined immunodeficiency, and Wiskott-Aldrich syndrome are two such conditions (although there are more). Infants and children with these diseases often have failure to thrive, life-threatening infections, severe viral infections, and/or severe diarrhea. Patients with Wiskott-Aldrich also have a bleeding disorder due to thrombocytopenia (low platelet counts and low platelet volumes—mean platelet volume). As a result, any infant or child with growth concerns, recurrent or severe infections, and eczema should be referred to a pediatric allergy/immunologist for evaluation of an underlying immunodeficiency.

There are many reasons why a referral to an allergist may help in the care of these patients. I have found a team approach between the patient, the family, the primary care provider, and the allergist most helpful. At our institution, a joint allergy and dermatology clinic also works quite well for our most severe patients. Families and patients need to be reminded that there is not one specific trigger or one way to manage.

Summary

I would recommend a referral to an allergist for the following:
- A patient with eczema on "exposed areas" (face, hands, and feet)
- A patient with diffuse eczema
- A patient with moderate-to-severe eczema
- A patient with escalating need for moderate-to high-potency topical steroids
- A patient with possible food allergy
- A patient with possible environmental (aeroallergen) trigger
- A patient with growth concerns or failure to thrive
- A patient with recurrent infections, severe infections, or difficult-to-treat infections
- A patient whose family is concerned about the role of allergies in his or her child's eczema

Suggested Readings

Caubet JC, PA Eigenmann. Allergic triggers in atopic dermatitis. *Immunol Allergy Clin North Am.* 2010;3(3):289-307.

Forbe LR, Saltzman RW, JM Spergel. Food allergies and atopic dermatitis: differentiating myth from reality. *Pediatr Ann.* 2008;38(2):84-90.

Sampson HA. The evaluation and management of food allergy in atopic dermatitis. *Clin Dermatol.* 2003;21(3):183-192.

SECTION V

INFECTIONS

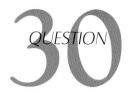

How Do I Treat Recalcitrant Warts?

Patrick McMahon, MD

Warts, or verrucae, are common viral infections of the skin and mucosal surfaces. They are caused by the human papilloma viruses (HPVs) of which there are over 100 types. Depending on the HPV type, warts favor different anatomical locations and can have varying morphologies. This brief review will highlight the various treatment modalities that can be used for the three main types of nongenital warts, namely common, flat, and plantar warts.

Most nongenital warts will eventually spontaneously resolve. Without treatment, spontaneous resolution was noted in approximately two-thirds of cases after 2 years.[1] However, warts can be emotionally troubling due to social embarrassment and painful, hindering physical activity. These are both justifiable indications for treatment. Keeping these indications in mind, if the patient is not bothered by his or her wart(s), the option of not treating should be offered. When treating, I tailor the therapy to the patient's age, immune status, the anatomic site of the wart, and the clinical morphology. Furthermore, therapies need to be consistent and all previous treatments that the patient has tried should be taken into consideration.

Two basic methods of treatment exist in treating warts: destructive therapies and immunotherapies. The goals of these therapies are to remove the wart, with the least amount of scarring, and to induce a lasting immunity. It should be noted that in patients with a decreased immune status, immunotherapies will be less effective. Of note many off label therapies will be discussed and their appropriateness, risks and benefits must be individualized to your patient.

Treating Common Warts (Verrucae Vulgaris)

Common warts can be found throughout the body but are predominately located on the hands, including the periungual location (Figures 30-1 and 30-2). I have found persistent patient-applied over-the-counter (OTC) therapies combined with intermittent office-based destructive therapy to be the most effective. Although this requires work

Figure 30-1. Multiple periungual warts on the fingers.

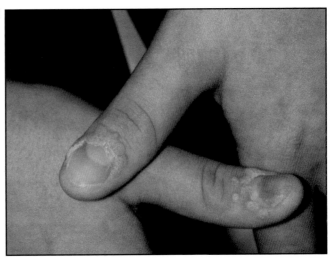

Figure 30-2. Thick verrucous papules on the palms.

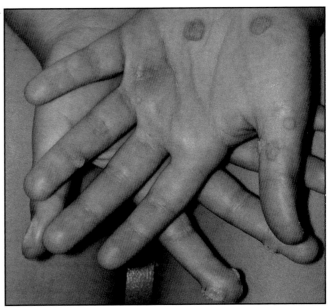

on behalf of the patient, and possibly his or her caretaker, I counsel him or her that a team-approach is the best way to achieve clearance. This can be best done by having the patient soak the affected area in water for 5 to 10 minutes daily, dry the area, and then apply an OTC salicylic acid formulation under occlusion. For younger children, soaking the area while bathing in a tub would be sufficient. Salicylic acid comes in several forms, including liquid, gel, plaster, pads, or roll-on sticks and can be found in varying percentages ranging from 6% to 40%. Choosing the best form will depend on the site and age of the child. In general, for thicker warts, a higher percentage salicylic acid will be needed. Occlusion can be achieved with a typical bandage or for frequently used areas, such as the fingers, several layers of tape. The occlusive dressing should be snug, but should not impede function. Salicylic acid should be avoided in any young or developmentally delayed children who may put the treated wart or bandage into their mouth. Alternatively, for a cheaper and simpler regimen, the patient can occlude the affected area with duct tape. Some have proposed that duct tape alone, left on for 6.5 days per week, can be effective[2]; however, the evidence for this monotherapy is slim and not convincing.[3,4] In between applications, the patient or parent should pare down the wart using an emery board or pumice stone, which should then be discarded because the wart virus will have been inoculated into it. If at any point this becomes painful or the area becomes macerated or bleeds, I counsel the patient to hold treatment for 3 to 4 days and then re-evaluate.

Ideally, the patient should be consistently seen in the office for treatment every 3 to 4 weeks. In-office treatment usually includes liquid nitrogen in the form of a spray gun or cotton-tipped applicator. The spray gun is faster, but can be fear inducing, especially in younger patients. Two thaws should be attempted, with the freezing generally lasting 5 seconds and each thaw lasting approximately 10 to 30 seconds. This time will depend on the thickness and diameter of the wart being treated. Paring down the wart is an essential part of the office-based therapy. This practice helps to thin the overlying callus to allow for better penetration of the liquid nitrogen into the viral-infected skin beneath. Treatment of the entire width of the wart is necessary to avoid persistence of the outer portion, an unwanted outcome known as a ring-wart. The goal of liquid nitrogen treatment is destruction of the wart by inducing a blister. Questioning the patient on subsequent visits as to whether or not a blister formed helps me adjust the duration of liquid nitrogen therapy. A blister usually forms 1 to 2 days after treatment and can be painful, depending on the body site. Once healed, the patient can commence with the at-home therapy discussed previously. Due to the pain induced by the blistering, anticipatory guidance is needed and holding treatment prior to scheduled events, such as sporting events, school examinations, or recitals, may be warranted. Another possible side effect of liquid nitrogen treatment, especially in pigmented individuals, is lightening of the skin upon healing (hypopigmentation). The above regimen should, therefore, be avoided in cosmetically sensitive areas, such as the face, especially in darkly pigmented patients. I advise the patient that several office treatments may be needed, typically 6 to 8, before resolution is achieved. If more treatment is needed, other more aggressive treatments are offered at that time (Table 30-1).

Treating Flat Warts (Verruca Planus)

Flat warts are often found on the face and dorsal hands of young patients (Figure 30-3). This type of wart has an increased tendency to spontaneously resolve. For these reasons, it is important to remember that any treatment should avoid scarring or pigmentary alterations. If these warts are bothersome to my patient, several topical treatments are available. Mild-strength salicylic acid is a treatment that a patient can obtain OTC. Many FDA approved medications are used off-label for warts and the appropriateness of their use should be tailored to your particular patient. Topical tretinoin cream or gel can be applied daily or twice daily. Starting with a mild potency, like 0.025% cream,

Table 30-1
Treatment of Warts

Treatment	Description
Salicylic acid under occlusion alone or combined with liquid nitrogen	First-line therapy for common and plantar warts Liquid nitrogen useful if child is able to tolerate procedure (see previous discussion for details)
Intralesional immunotherapy	*Candida* antigen injected directly into wart to stimulate local immune response Useful for common and plantar warts (Mumps antigen also used)
Topical retinoid	Cream or gel can be useful for flat warts, especially on face where destructive therapies are best avoided (see discussion on flat warts)
Laser therapy	Pulsed-dye laser most commonly used Useful for isolated or few warts in older children able to tolerate the procedure Carbon-dioxide and frequency-double Nd:YAG lasers are ablative and scarring
Cimetidine	Low efficacy Evidence in literature is conflicting[4] Dose 30 to 40 mg/kg/d divided tid or qid
Topical cantharidin	Blistering agent No longer available in the United States Solutions of 0.7% or 1% available from Canada Apply small amount of liquid to entire wart in office, cover with a bandage, and have patient wash liquid off in 4 to 8 hours Repeat treatment every 2 to 3 weeks

ND:YAG indicates neodymium-doped yttrium aluminum garnet

is best with the goal of inducing only mild erythema of the affected area. Tazarotene 0.05% cream or gel is another alternative. Imiquimod 5% cream daily can be used alone or in addition to a topical tretinoin therapy; however, there is limited evidence for this expensive option.[4] Similarly, 5-fluorouracil 5% cream twice daily is listed as a treatment option for flat warts; however, once again evidence of its efficacy is limited and this is chemotherapy whose safety is unknown in children.[4] I generally avoid using liquid nitrogen for facial flat warts, especially in patients with dark skin given the possibility for lightening of the skin. For flat warts on the dorsal hands of patients with lighter skin, light freezing with liquid nitrogen is a feasible option. Other more aggressive treatments for flat warts are less practical in a pediatric population and include laser treatment or electrodessication.

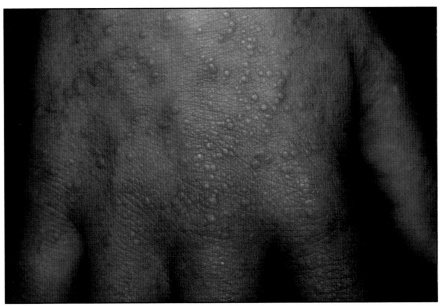

Figure 30-3. Many flat warts on the dorsal hand.

Treating Plantar Warts (Verruca Plantaris)

Plantar warts tend to be the most refractory and unfortunately, the most painful. As a first-line therapy, salicylic acid is still a good option. Utilizing the tips from the above section on treating common warts can be helpful. Due to the thick skin of the soles, a stronger salicylic acid preparation is best, such as a 40% patch that can be applied directly to the wart every day or every other day. In between applications, soaking the foot in water and paring down the wart can help alleviate the pain caused by the overlying callus, as well as allow for better penetration of the salicylic acid. Liquid nitrogen therapy is a useful, albeit painful, adjunct to this at-home regimen. Plantar warts may require longer freeze-thaw times due to thicker stratum corneum. Topical application of cantharidin can be used to induce blistering of plantar warts. This product is commonly used but not FDA approved and is currently not available in the United States but can be obtained from Canada as a solution of 0.7% or 1%.

A small amount of the liquid can be applied in the office to the entire wart surface with the wooden edge of an applicator stick. Allow the liquid to dry and then cover with a bandage. Have the patient remove the bandage and wash the area 4 to 6 hours after application. This treatment is painless; however, the goal is to create a blister that itself can produce pain. This treatment can be repeated every 2 to 3 weeks and if no blistering was produced initially, the patient can be instructed to leave the solution on for a longer period of time, up to 12 hours. Avoid applying this blistering agent to folds as severe burns have been caused by inadvertent spread in such areas. Lastly, developing a "ring-wart" is a potential untoward outcome of this treatment if the entire wart is not treated and the periphery persists after blistering occurs centrally. Given the refractory nature of plantar warts, if persistent pain is experienced despite the above regimens, intralesional immunotherapy therapy can be tried but is off label (see Table 30-1). *Candida albicans* antigen intralesional injection is the most common agent used and can be done so monthly by injecting 0.1 to 0.3 mL of the test antigen directly into each wart. I initiate treatment with a solution diluted with normal saline to a concentration of 1:100 or 1:50 (*Candida* antigen:saline), increasing the concentration to 1:10 on future applications if needed depending on the outcome. A total of up to 1 mL of the solution can be used per treatment depending on how many warts are being treated. Lastly, upon referral to a specialist laser therapies are more aggressive treatments that may be utilized in patients old enough to tolerate these procedures. If scarring methods are explored, such as CO_2 laser or surgical excision, the patient should be counseled that the plantar scar produced may be painful itself and cure from the wart is still not guaranteed. Therefore, these more permanent therapies should be reserved as a last resort.[5]

Immunocompromised Patients and Warts

Importantly, remember that in immunosuppressed patients, warts are more common, have varying clinical appearances, and can be particularly widespread and recalcitrant. This population includes those patients on immunosuppressive medications, HIV-infected individuals, leukemia/lymphoma patients, and those with congenital immunodeficiencies. There are also newly described genetic syndromes that include extensive verruca as part of their phenotype, namely WHIM syndrome (warts, hypogammaglobulinemia, infections, and myelokathexis) and combined immunodeficiency with a mutation in the DOCK8 gene. Keeping this in mind is helpful as your approach may be more aggressive from the outset and expectations can be adjusted accordingly. Furthermore, having widespread or extremely persistent warts can at times be the sign of a previously undiagnosed immunocompromised state.

Summary

Even though there are several treatments discussed, it is important to note that the evidence for many treatments is lacking. In a 2006 Cochrane Review of the topical treatments for cutaneous warts, it was concluded that although there was a general "lack of evidence," overall salicylic acid appeared to "have a therapeutic effect" over placebo and no other topical treatment was found to have a higher cure rate.[4] This review was republished in 2009 without any change to the conclusion. The treatment of warts can be arduous and frustrating for the patient, caretaker, and practitioner. Since some of the treatments can be painful, it is important in the pediatric population to discuss the treatment options, including the risks, openly with the patient and caretaker. As warts are benign and eventually self-limited, remember to always discuss the option of patiently waiting for spontaneous resolution.

References

1. Massing AM, Epstein WL. Natural history of warts. A two-year study. *Arch Dermatol.* 1963;87:306-310.
2. Abernethy H, Cho C, DeLanoy A, et al. Clinical inquiries. What nonpharmacological treatments are effective against common nongenital warts? *J Fam Pract.* 2006;55(9):801-802.

3. Wenner R, Askari SK, Cham PM, Kedrowski DA, Liu A, Warshaw EM. Duct tape for the treatment of common warts in adults: a double-blind randomized controlled trial. *Arch Dermatol.* 2007;143(3):309-313.
4. Gibbs S, Harvey I. Topical treatments for cutaneous warts. *Cochrane Database Syst Rev.* 2006;3:CD001781.
5. James WD, Berger T, Elston MD. *Andrew's Diseases of the Skin: Clinical Dermatology.* 10th ed. Philadelphia, PA: W.B. Saunders; 2006:404-413.

WHEN SHOULD I EXPECT PROPERLY TREATED TINEA CAPITIS TO IMPROVE? WHAT OTHER TREATMENT OPTIONS ARE AVAILABLE WHEN GRISEOFULVIN FAILS?

Sheila F. Friedlander, MD

Tinea capitis is a very clever disorder as it can masquerade as dandruff (seborrheic dermatitis) or folliculitis and is even sometimes mistaken for a bacterial abscess when it presents with pustules or as a kerion (Figures 31-1 to 31-3). I always utilize griseofulvin (FDA approved for children 2 years and above) when I believe the infection is caused by *Microsporum canis* (*M canis*) (transmitted from an infected cat or dog), which responds best to high-dose griseofulvin.[1] However, I more commonly empirically initiate treatment with terbinafine because more than 90% of North American tinea capitis is caused by *Trichophyton tonsurans* (*T tonsurans*), which generally responds nicely to terbinafine within 4 weeks (This drug is FDA approved for age 4 years and above.). There is no consensus "best treatment" for dermatophyte scalp infections caused by *T tonsurans*; however, many experts feel that terbinafine and other newer agents may lead to more rapid response.[2,3]

If you prefer to use griseofulvin for everyone, start with 20 mg/kg/day microsize taken with a fatty food such as whole milk, and expect to treat for at least 6 to 8 weeks. With terbinafine, you can usually treat for 4 weeks, utilizing 5 to 7 mg/kg/day, rounded to the most convenient percentage of a full 250-mg-sized tablet (eg, ¼, ½, or full tablet) not to exceed one tablet (250 mg) a day. Terbinafine can be purchased very inexpensively in 250-mg-sized tablet form at large pharmacies. The pills can be split as needed and put in pudding or peanut butter. The granule form of terbinafine is quite expensive and hard to find, and most kids will do just fine with the tablets. If a child cannot swallow pills, he or she can be prescribed liquid griseofulvin (125 mg/5 ml).

You should expect some response within 2 to 4 weeks (scale and redness decreased). Do not, however, expect hair to regrow for several months. Your patient may not be completely clear but particularly with kerions you should see some decrease in inflammation.

Figure 31-1. Tinea capitis with scaly plaque and localized kerion.

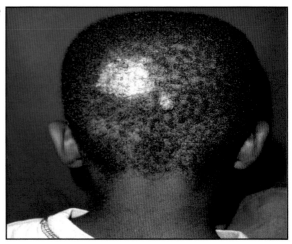

Figure 31-2. Tinea capitis kerion and localized plaque.

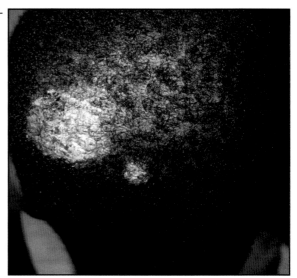

Figure 31-3. Tinea capitis in 2 siblings, note postauricular lymphadenopathy in the eldest.

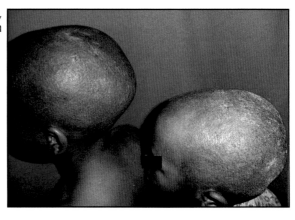

If a kerion has not improved within 2 weeks, some experts will add prednisone 1 mg/kg for 7 to 10 days. If classic tinea has not responded within 4 weeks, check for noncompliance (are they taking griseofulvin with food?) and make sure they are using a topical antifungal such as selenium sulfide or ketoconazole shampoo. Make sure there is not another infected person (or animal!) in close contact with the patient.

If all of the above is in order and the patient shows no improvement after 1 month, I would check to see what organism grew out (thus the need to obtain culture initially). If you are dealing with *M canis*, realize that it may take a while to see improvement and consider increasing the griseofulvin dose to 25 mg/kg/day. If you are dealing with *T tonsurans*, make sure your dose of terbinafine is reasonable (at least 6 mg/kg/day); if it is, and you are dealing with a *Trichophyton* species, you can hang in there for a few more weeks, or consider a switch to itraconazole, fluconazole, or griseofulvin. Unfortunately, published cure rates with these drugs are not better for *T tonsurans*, but after 1 month most families are anxious for a change.

Regarding laboratory tests, any patient on any therapy for more than 8 weeks gets liver function test (LFT) evaluation in our office. Regarding terbinafine, baseline LFTs as well as complete blood count and repeated LFTs if treatment longer 6 weeks are recommended, but some experts will make certain the patients have no underlying disorders and opt to obtain laboratories only if the patient develops symptoms. I would not use terbinafine on any patient with underlying liver disease. I warn the family of treated patients of possible side effects such as hives and rare risks of liver disease.

References

1. Lipozencic J, Skerlev M, Orofino-Costa R, et al.; Tinea Capitis Study Group. A randomized, double-blind, parallel-group, duration-finding study of oral terbinafine and open-label, high-dose griseofulvin in children with tinea capitis due to *Microsporum* species. *Br J Dermatol*. 2002;146(5):816-823.
2. González U, Seaton T, Bergus G, Jacobson J, Martínez-Monzón C. Systemic antifungal therapy for tinea capitis in children. *Cochrane Database Syst Rev*. 2007;(4):CD004685.
3. Elewski BE, Cáceres HW, DeLeon L, et al. Terbinafine hydrochloride oral granules versus oral griseofulvin suspension in children with tinea capitis: results of two randomized, investigator-blinded, multicenter, international, controlled trials. *J Am Acad Dermatol*. 2008;59(1):41-54. Epub 2008 Apr 18.

HOW DO I MANAGE AND HELP PATIENTS PREVENT RECURRENT METHICILLIN-RESISTANT STAPHYLOCOCCUS AUREUS FURUNCULOSIS?

Sheila F. Friedlander, MD

Cutaneous methicillin-resistant *Staphylococcus aureus* (MRSA) infections are growing problem for practitioners (Figure 32-1). In the last decade, an increasing number of community-acquired forms of MRSA have been noted, which now accounts for the majority of recurrent furunculosis we see.[1] When these infections are recurrent, more investigative work and effort are required. It is always important to get a good history including family and social history: Does anyone work in a hospital or health care facility? Does anyone else have recurrent boils or skin lesions?

It is a good idea to review basic preventive messages, which include (1) keep draining wounds covered; (2) attention to personal hygiene with regular bathing and washing of hands with soaps or alcohol-based gels; and (3) no sharing of personal items such as towels, razors, and pillowcases/linens.

If your patient has recurrent infections, you want to be sure of the nature of his or her organism; is it definitely *S aureus*, and has a D-test been performed to check for inducible clindamycin resistance? Has he or she been compliant with therapy? Does he or she have a chronic pruritic dermatitis (atopic dermatitis, scabies), diabetes, an immunodeficiency, or some other disorder predisposing him or her to recurrent infection? If he or she has eczema, has everything been done to get it under good control?

The optimal therapy for recurrent MRSA infections includes the following:
- Incise and drain (I&D) of a simple abscess or boil. This may be sufficient therapy if an isolated small (<5 cm) lesion is present.
- Antibiotic therapy is recommended for severe or extensive disease, multiple sites of infection, very young children, and anyone who looks sick or has rapidly progressive findings.

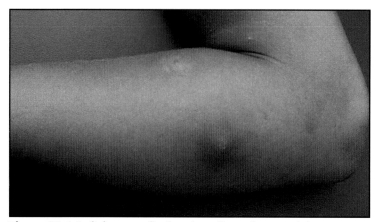

Figure 32-1. Left forearm fluctuant erythematous nodule.

- Oral clindamycin or trimethoprim (TMP)-sulfamethoxazole (SMX) (TMP/SMX only indicated if over 2 months of age) are options for *aureus*; if streptococcal infection is a concern, TMP/SMX is not a good choice.
- Tetracyclines such as doxycycline or minocycline are options in older children but should not be used in children less than 8 years of age and do not reliably cover streptococcal infection.

According to recent guidelines published by the Infectious Diseases Society of America,[1-3] decolonization can be considered in the following situations:

1. Recurrent infections occur despite optimal wound care and hygiene measures.
2. Ongoing transmission is occurring within the household or close contacts.

There is no universally successful decolonization plan for eradication of recurrent staph infections. However, some steps are commonly utilized. Nasal mupirocin twice daily for 5 to 10 days in combination with or without antiseptic agents, such as chlorhexidine for 5 to 14 days, have been utilized. Many people now recommend twice weekly 15-minute dilute bleach baths for approximately 3 months. One-half teaspoon of household bleach per gallon of water, or half cup per full tub (40 gallons of water) is the usual concentration recommended.

Oral antibiotics should only be used for active infection. Some providers will add oral rifampin to the primary antibiotic if infections recur despite the above interventions.

The possibility of a nidus of colonization or infection within the family or a close contact should be considered. All close contacts and family members should adhere to the hygiene measures already mentioned. They should be evaluated for evidence of *S aureus* infection. If the index patient has recurrent infections, family members and close contacts should be evaluated for evidence of *S aureus* infection. If someone is infected, they should be treated and decolonization strategies considered for that individual. Nasal and topical body decolonization of asymptomatic household contacts can be considered.

Routine screening cultures prior to decolonization are not necessary if at least one of the prior infections was documented to be MRSA. Surveillance cultures are not routinely recommended.

References

1. Larsen AR, Stegger M, Böcher S, Sørum M, Monnet DL, Skov RL. Emergence and characterization of community-associated methicillin-resistant *Staphyloccocus aureus* infections in Denmark, 1999 to 2006. *J Clin Microbiol.* 2009;47(1):73-78. Epub 2008 Oct 29.
2. Liu C, Bayer A, Cosgrove SE, et al. Clinical practice guidelines by the Infectious Diseases Society of America for the treatment of methicillin-resistant *Staphylococcus aureus* infections in adults and children: executive summary. *Clin Infect Dis.* 2011;52(3):285-292.
3. Liu C, Bayer A, Cosgrove SE, et al. Clinical practice guidelines by the Infectious Diseases Society of America for the treatment of methicillin-resistant *Staphylococcus aureus* infections in adults and children. *Clin Infect Dis.* 2011;52(3):e18-e55.

HOW DO I MANAGE RECALCITRANT HEAD LICE?

Dirk M. Elston, MD

Head louse resistance is becoming widespread. Permethrin resistance was reported in Israel in 1994 but is now widespread in the United States, Europe, and Asia. Assays for genetic mutations, including the common T929I and L932F mutations, have shown that the majority of lice in many communities are now resistant to permethrin. Cross-resistance among pyrethroids is common, and alternative pyrethroid preparations add little to our existing armamentarium. Although many apparent treatment failures are from inadequate therapy or re-infestation, what is the clinician to do when faced with truely resistant lice?

Prescription Therapy

The good news is that a highly effective, non-neurotoxic agent based on benzyl alcohol is now commercially available. Marketed under the brand name Ulesfia, this agent represents a significant improvement in the way we treat head lice, and it is my first choice for the treatment of head lice. Benzyl alcohol can cause mast cell degranulation, so the product may cause scalp itching, but it is generally very well tolerated. Given concerns about a possible link between permethrin and childhood leukemia, benzyl alcohol is now considered by many to be the agent of choice for the treatment of head lice.

Natroba topical suspension is a new entry into the market that contains spinosad as well as benzyl alcohol. It is indicated for the treatment of head lice in patients 4 years and older. Spinosad is a mixture of spinosyn A and spinosyn D in a 5 to 1 ratio. Spinosad is derived from the soil actinomycete *Saccharopolyspora spinosa*. It causes neuronal excitation, paralysis, and death in insects and is best regarded as a "naturally derived insecticide." When a neurotoxic agent is required because of lack of efficacy or intolerance to alternatives, permethrin is seldom justified, given the widespread prevalence of resistance. In contrast, malathion (not recommended for children under 6 years) resistance appears to be relatively uncommon in the United States, although it is more common in Europe. Even when product labeling suggests a single application, evidence suggests that a second application at 10 days is prudent with many agents, and that the 10-day interval is superior to a 1-week interval. Agents such as carbaryl and pirimiphos often remain active in the face of pyrethroid resistance, but they are not readily available in the United States. In Britain, double resistance to permethrin and malathion is becoming increasingly common.

Ivermectin has been used off-label for head lice, both as a topical agent and orally at a dose of 200 mcg per kg in children over 5 years of age, but concerns about potential neurologic toxicity have limited its use to date. Some have advocated the use of oral trim-ethoprim/sulfamethoxazole (TMP-SMZ) for the treatment of head lice, but a recent study showed that lindane plus TMP-SMZ was no better than lindane alone and it may prove to be no better than placebo. Piperonal has been used as a pediculicide and louse repellent in Europe. It is not available in the United States. Essential oils have been shown to have some efficacy against lice and are aggressively marketed through the Internet, but these agents are potential contact allergens.

Nonprescription Therapy

Shaving of all parasitized hair will eradicate head lice but is not acceptable in many societies. While dilute solutions of vinegar or formic acid are not capable of dissolving nit cement, they cause flattening of the hair cuticle and can make combing easier. Hair con-ditioners can also be used. Many pediculicides come with a plastic nit comb, but they are prone to break, especially in children with curly hair. Metal nit combs are available at some stores and through the Internet but are relatively expensive. Battery-powered electrified combs are quite expensive and are seldom necessary. I find that their main attraction is the noise and flashing lights that suggest they are doing something spectacular.

Hot air devices, including blow driers and the Louse Buster system, require at least 30 minutes to desiccate lice, and many children resist the procedure. Cetaphil Gentle Skin Cleanser and a blow dryer were reported to be effective in one study, but this requires further validation. Dimethicone can occlude respiratory passages of the louse, but without the addition of benzyl alcohol, the respiratory spiracles close when the louse become wet. Wet combing has limited efficacy unless done thoroughly and repeatedly, an arduous task.

Decontamination and Prevention

Machine laundering should be used to decontaminate washable hats, scarves, linens, and other fomites. Either washing with a water temperature of at least 50°C or thorough drying is effective.

Contact with untreated classmates may result in apparent treatment failure in the absence of drug resistance. Classroom and community education about the signs of louse infestation and options for treatment is mandatory. Routine screening of school children by the school nurse can detect louse infestation before it spreads widely through the school (Figures 33-1 and 33-2). Except in very humid climates, nits more than ¼ inch from the scalp are not reliable evidence of active infestation. While some authors have suggest-ed that louse screening is demeaning to children, my experience is that the children read-ily accept it as a fact of life. Personally, I would find infestation to be the more demeaning

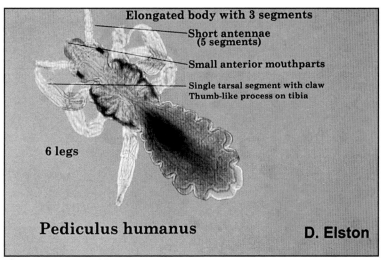

Figure 33-1. Head louse.

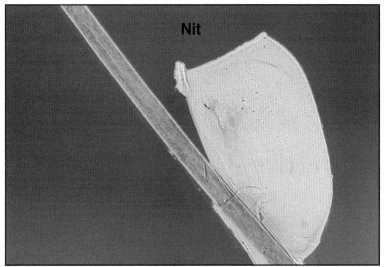

Figure 33-2. Nit attached to a hair shaft.

of the two. Simple measures can be instituted to reduce the spread of lice between classmates. Hats, scarves, and jackets should be stored separately under each student's desk, rather than in a pile at the bottom of the closet. While I support routine screening, "no-nit" policies have never been shown to reduce the spread of lice, but exclude many children from the classroom unnecessarily. Such policies should be eliminated.

Suggested Readings

Ameen M, Arenas R, Villanueva-Reyes J, et al. Oral ivermectin for treatment of pediculosis capitis. *Pediatr Infect Dis J.* 2010;29:991-993.

Borkhardt A, Wilda M, Fuchs U, Gortner L, Reiss I. Congenital leukaemia after heavy abuse of permethrin during pregnancy. *Arch Dis Child Fetal Neonatal Ed.* 2003;88(5):F436-F4367.

Frankowski BL, Bocchini JA Jr; Council on School Health and Committee on Infectious Diseases. Head lice. *Pediatrics*. 2010;126(2):392-403.

Menegaux F, Baruchel A, Bertrand Y, et al. Household exposure to pesticides and risk of childhood acute leukaemia. *Occup Environ Med*. 2006;63(2):131-134.

Rutman H. Ivermectin versus malathion for head lice. *N Engl J Med*. 2010;362(25):2426-2427.

The images were produced while the author was a full-time federal employee. They are in the public domain.

What Is Molluscum contagiosum and How Is It Treated?

Lisa Arkin, MD

Background

Molluscum contagiosum (MC) is a common cutaneous viral infection characterized by discrete flesh-colored, monomorphic-appearing umbilicated papules. It commonly affects the skin but can also involve the mucus membranes. In immunocompetent patients, its course is generally benign and self-limited, with most patients spontaneously clearing in 6 to 9 months without treatment. The morbidity is primarily aesthetic or due to mild associated symptoms; most patients seek treatment due to concern about spreading the disease to others.

The virus is classified in the *Poxviridae* family and 4 genetically distinct but clinically indistinguishable subtypes (molluscum contagiosum virus [MCV] I–IV) have been identified. In the United States, 98% of infections appear to result from MCV-I. MCV-II infection is more common among patients with human immunodeficiency virus (HIV), while MCV-III and IV infections are extremely rare. Because the virus requires cell-mediated immunity for clearance, patients with T-cell dysfunction are at increased risk for developing severe disease. In particular, those with HIV may have widespread, persistent infection with atypical features. A low CD4 count increases the risk of extensive facial involvement, which may resemble cutaneous cryptococcosis, and increases the risk of bacterial superinfection. In addition, due to decreased cell-mediated immunity from a predominantly TH2-skewed axis, patients with poorly controlled atopic dermatitis are at increased risk for MC and other cutaneous viral infections including herpes simplex virus. These patients have been reported to develop larger MC lesions with more widespread anatomic involvement.

Figure 34-1. Flesh-colored umbilicated papules consistent with MC.

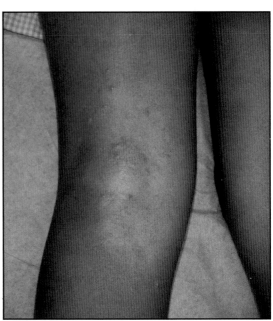

Epidemiology

The virus is spread by direct skin-to-skin contact or via fomites including gymnasium equipment, benches, and towels. In children, lesions may occur anywhere but most commonly involve the trunk and extremities. This is in contrast to adults, where the infection is more likely to be sexually transmitted and localized to the abdomen, genitals, and medial thighs.

The largest epidemiologic study of pediatric dermatology patients with MC infection found that two-thirds were younger than 8 years of age. Boys and girls were equally affected across all age groups, and most patients were otherwise healthy. The trunk was the most frequently reported location while the face was rarely affected. Half of patients presented with fewer than 15 lesions distributed in more than one anatomic region. One-quarter of patients were concomitantly diagnosed with atopic dermatitis. In contrast to prior studies, this investigation found no correlation between underlying atopic dermatitis and increased severity of MC infection.

Clinical Presentation

The diagnosis is predominantly a clinical one made on the basis of characteristic morphology. Lesions appear as small, pearly-white or flesh-colored, dome-shaped papules with central umbilication (Figure 34-1). They are typically restricted to the skin but rarely may involve mucosal surfaces, most commonly the genital mucosa or conjunctiva. In addition, 10% to 30% of patients have been reported to develop an eczematous dermatitis associated with the infection, which can be quite pruritic and increases the risk of autoinoculation due to scratching. Patients who are febrile, have widespread disease with greater than 50 lesions, or are refractory to treatment should raise suspicion for a missed diagnosis or underlying immunodeficiency.

Table 34-1
Treatment for Molluscum Contagiosum

- Destructive measures
  - Cryotherapy
  - Curettage
  - Cantharidin
- Immunomodulators
  - Topical imiquimod
  - Cimetidine
- Vitamin A derivatives
  - Tretinoin
  - Adapalene
- Antiviral agents (for HIV)
  - HAART
  - Topical cidofovir

HAART indicates highly active antiretroviral therapy; HIV, human immunodeficiency virus

---

Treatment

A recent Cochrane review found that no single intervention was convincingly effective in the treatment of MC. Since most patients will eventually clear the infection spontaneously, benign neglect is an acceptable choice for patients and families (Table 34-1).

For patients who seek treatment, destructive measures are commonly employed. Cryotherapy and curettage are fairly effective but limited by pain and discomfort. Cantharidin, an extract from the blister beetle, is a non-FDA approved phosphodiesterase inhibitor that induces blistering and extrusion of the virus in treated lesions. The largest retrospective chart review of children treated with cantharidin found that 98% of patients cleared or experienced significant improvement. Side effects including pain, erythema, or pruritus at sites of blistering were mild and transient. Nearly all parents reported that they would proceed with cantharidin treatment again. In spite of this and other studies supporting its safe and effective use, cantharidin has become increasingly difficult to obtain due to persistent FDA concerns regarding its safety. Many offices no longer have access to the agent, and it remains to be seen whether cantharidin will become obsolete in the treatment of this disease.

There is some evidence to support the use of immunomodulatory agents including topical imiquimod, a toll-like receptor-7 agonist that amplifies the innate and adaptive immune response to viral infection. Several small randomized, controlled trials have demonstrated resolution of MC lesions after application of topical imiquimod 5 times per week for 4 to 6 weeks but other trials have failed to prove efficacy. In addition, anecdotal reports have supported the use of other immunomodulators including cimetidine. There is also limited evidence for the utility of retinoids, which may be applied beginning every other day and advancing to twice daily for 4 to 6 weeks.

For patients with HIV and acquired immunodeficiency syndrome, highly active anti-retroviral therapy is the treatment of choice. These drugs promote clearance of the infection by improving T-cell function and decreasing HIV viral load. Cidofovir, a nucleoside analog with broad activity against DNA viruses, can also be used topically and is a useful adjuvant for refractory MC in patients with HIV.

Finally, gentle skin care is recommended for all patients. To reduce disease transmission, patients should be instructed to abstain from community swimming pools as well as sharing towels or athletic equipment.

Suggested Readings

Agromayor M, Ortiz P, Lopez-Estebaranz IL, Gonzalez-Nicolas J, Esteban M, Martin-Gallardo A. Molecular epidemiology of molluscum contagiosum virus and analysis of the host-serum antibody response in Spanish HIV-negative patients. *J Med Virol.* 2002;66(2):151-158.

Al-Mutairi N, Al-Doukhi A, Al-Farag S, Al-Haddad A. Comparative study on the efficacy, safety and acceptability of imiquimod 5% cream versus cryotherapy for molluscum contagiosum in children. *Pediatr Dermatol.* 2010;27(4): 388-394.

Brown J, Janniger CK, Schwartz RA, Silverberg NB. Childhood molluscum contagiosum. *Int J Dermatol.* 2006; 45(2):93-99.

Dohill MA, Lin P, Lee J, Lucky AW, Paller AS, Eichenfield LF. The epidemiology of molluscum contagiosum in children. *J Am Acad Dermatol.* 2006;54(1):47-54.

Otto A. FDA said to be blocking cantharidin importation. *Skin Allergy News.* 2010;41(12):6. http://www.nxtbook. com/nxtbooks/elsevier/san_201012/index.php?startid=6#/6

Sampson HA. Atopic dermatitis: immunologic mechanisms in relationship to phenotype. *Pediatr Allergy Immunol.* 2001;12(Suppl 14):62-68.

Silverberg N, Sidbury R, Mancini AJ. Childhood molluscum contagiosum: experience with cantharidin therapy in 300 patients. *J Am Acad Dermatol.* 2000;43(3):503-537.

van der Wouden JC, van der Sande R, van Suijlekom-Smit LW, Berger M, Butler C, Koning S. Interventions for cutaneous molluscum contagiosum. *Cochrane Database Syst Rev.* 2009;(4):CD004767.

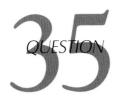

SHOULD I TREAT RECURRENT HERPES SIMPLEX ON THE LIP?

John C. Browning, MD, FAAD, FAAP

Cold sores, also known as herpes labialis, are recurrent blisters that appear on the lips. They are often brought on by an upper respiratory infection, which is why they are called "cold" sores. Stress, sunlight, or anything that impairs the cutaneous immune system can also cause an outbreak. Most patients have about two episodes a year but they can recur every few weeks.

Herpes labialis is caused by the herpes simplex virus (HSV). Usually HSV-1 is associated with herpes labialis and HSV-2 is associated with genital herpes. However, in patients who have engaged in oral-genital sex, HSV-2 can infect the lips and HSV-1 the genitalia.

Initial infection is usually characterized by multiple painful blisters on the inside and outside of the mouth. Recurrent infections are characterized by clustered vesicles on the lip. Recurrences occur because the virus lies dormant in the dorsal root ganglion and ascends during times of low immunity. Patients usually complain of burning or tingling 1 to 2 days before the vesicles appear. The vesicles become purulent and then crust over as they heal. It usually takes 7 to 14 days from initial outbreak to complete healing.

Diagnosis can often be established by history and physical examination. Tzanck smear, direct fluorescence antibody, polymerase chain reaction, or herpes viral culture can confirm the diagnosis.

Treatment is not indicated in most cases of herpes labialis. The lesions will crust over and self-resolve.

Treatment may be indicated in the following cases:
- Herpes labialis occurring more than 6 times a year
  - Treatment may be pursued in these cases because patients are tired of having visible sores more than a few times a year.
- Prolonged episodes of herpes labialis
  - Usually herpes labialis lasts 1 to 2 weeks but in some people it can last longer and this could be a problem for them with work and social interactions.

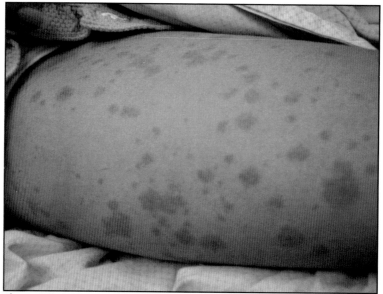

Figure 35-1. Herpes-associated EM.

- Association of erythema multiforme (EM) with HSV outbreak (Figure 35-1)
  - Eighty percent of recurrent cases of EM are associated with HSV infection. Affected individuals have a unique immune response to HSV, which leads to EM with every outbreak of HSV. The rash of EM is characterized by multiple targetoid papules on the trunk and extremities. It can be of great cosmetic concern due to the stigma of having a prolonged and unusual rash. EM usually evolves over 1 to 2 weeks and then takes 2 to 3 weeks to resolve. Fever and mouth sores can occur in some cases of EM.
  - EM cannot be treated with antivirals but suppressive antiviral therapy can prevent HSV infection, which can trigger EM.
- Being in a high-risk situation
  - New baby at home
    - HSV can cause a fatal encephalitis and hepatitis in neonates.
  - Day care or nursery worker
    - They can pass HSV to infants, which can be fatal.
  - Health care provider
    - Those working in nurseries, bone marrow transplant units, or intensive care units may want to consider treatment.
  - Close contact with immunocompromised individuals
    - Some immunocompromised individuals are at risk for invasive HSV.
  - Being around family members or co-workers with impaired skin barriers, such as atopic dermatitis or ichthyosis

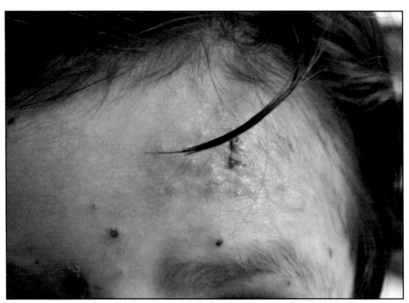

Figure 35-2. Active herpes simplex infection on the forehead.

- ▪ Individuals with impaired skin barriers can develop Kaposi varicelliform eruption. This is called eczema herpeticum when it affects those with atopic dermatitis. It is a disseminated cutaneous HSV infection characterized by multiple superficial vesicles and painful punched-out erosions all over the body (Figure 35-2). Often the patients have fever and look toxic and can become superinfected with bacteria, which can lead to sepsis. Ophthalmology evaluation should be pursued when involvement of the eyes occurs.
- ○ Extensive pain or discomfort associated with the outbreak
  - ▪ Some patients complain of a greater degree of discomfort with infection and would benefit from prompt, early treatment.
- ○ Having a job in which a visible cold sore could pose a problem
  - ▪ Examples might include being a model, actor, or television reporter.
- ○ Certain athletes
  - ▪ Wrestlers and other athletes who engage in contact sports are at high risk for passing HSV to other players. The National Collegiate Athletic Association requires a minimum of 120 hours from the start of therapy until an athlete can resume competition.

When given during the prodromal period after the start of burning or tingling, systemic therapy can often halt further progression and outbreak of the vesicles. Chronic suppressive therapy is often used when more than six outbreaks occur a year. Recurrences may be noted more commonly in areas that are exposed to sun (such as the lower lip) and sun protection may help prevent flares.

Often the treatment of recurrent HSV is a personal choice. It needs to be made in conjunction with the child and parent and is based on many different factors. Hand washing should always be advocated, as should avoidance of kissing and sharing beverages or utensils.

Suggested Readings

Fatahzadeh M, Schwartz RA. Human herpes simplex labialis. *Clin Exp Dermatol.* 2007;32(6):625-630.

Fatahzadeh M, Schwartz RA. Human herpes simplex virus infections: epidemiology, pathogenesis, symptomatology, diagnosis, and management. *J Am Acad Dermatol.* 2007;57(5):737-763; quiz 764-766.

St Pierre SA, Bartlett BL, Schlosser BJ. Practical management measures for patients with recurrent herpes labialis. *Skin Therapy Lett.* 2009;14(8):1-3.

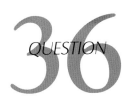

36

When Should Warts Be Treated?

Albert C. Yan, MD, FAAP, FAAD

Background

Warts are caused by infection of epidermal keratinocytes by human papillomavirus. Depending on the strain and the site of infection, warts can present as small flat-topped papules (flat warts or verruca plana often seen on the face or extremities), thick keratotic papules (common or plantar warts, which can be found at any site, but especially the extremities), clustered keratotic spires (filiform or digitate warts most often found on the face or scalp), and soft often grouped papules or papillomatous lesions in the genital area (condyloma acuminata).

About two-thirds of common warts will have spontaneously resolved within 2 years of onset. Active nonintervention may be reasonable consideration. However, in the interim, warts may warrant therapy for a few reasons:

- Warts may spread to other sites.
- Warts may become symptomatic when present at certain anatomic sites (such as the soles of the feet, the perianal area, or the hands).
- Warts may be stigmatizing (especially when they are present on the face, hands, or knees; Figure 36-1).
- Children, their family members, or other household contacts who are immunocompromised may be at risk for more exuberant involvement so treatment may prevent large and widespread warts.
- Children with disrupted skin barriers as might be seen in those with atopic dermatitis may also be at risk for more widespread disease.

For these reasons, patients and their parents may seek treatment for warts.

Treatment depends in part on the site of involvement and the types of warts being treated. Most children prefer to avoid painful treatment options where possible, although older children and adolescents may be willing to tolerate painful destructive modalities for more rapid resolution of the warts.

Figure 36-1. Filiform wart on the lower lip.

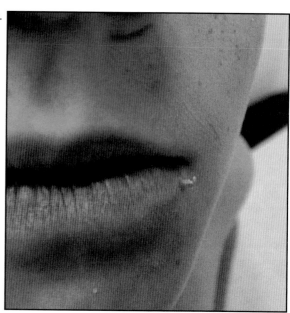

Figure 36-2. Thick hyperkeratotic plaque of warts with punctate hemorrhage on the heel.

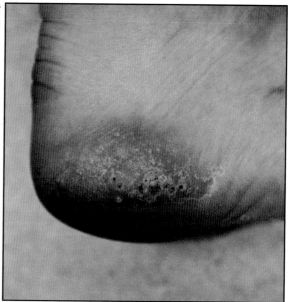

Common and Plantar Warts

These usually occur on thickly keratinized surfaces such as the skin of the extremities (Figure 36-2).

Randomized controlled trials and the Cochrane analysis of studies have indicated that topical salicylic acid preparations are an effective means of treating warts. Salicylic acid is also a relatively painless therapy. However, some patience is required with its use since it may take several weeks of consistent application for the warts to resolve.

In clinical practice, patients are advised to soak the affected area in warm water (at about 110°F) for between 1 and 5 minutes, since there is some evidence to suggest that heat alone can hasten resolution of warts. The soaking also improves penetration of the topically applied 17% salicylic acid. Once the material dries, the warts can be occluded using waterproof tape such as that found in local pharmacies or duct tape. The tape is left overnight or until the next evening as tolerated. Once the tape is removed, a dedicated pumice stone or nail file can be used to débride the wart surface. This procedure can be repeated nightly until the warts resolve. If significant irritation arises, a 1 to 2 day break can be recommended and then treatment can be restarted once the irritation subsides.

Other topical agents that may have some benefit from anecdotal reports include trials of topical imiquimod cream and topical sinecatechins ointment. Both are indicated for treatment of external genital warts in adults but would be an off-label indication for common warts, imiquimod as a once daily on Mondays, Wednesdays, and Fridays or sinecatechins as a 1 to 3 times daily treatment.

If insufficient response is seen despite good adherence to this regimen, cryotherapy can be considered using either a commercially available volatile compressed gas (such as diethyl propane or similar product, including products such as VerrucaFreeze [CryoSurgery, Inc, Nashville, TN] www.cryosurgeryinc.com). We do not want them to just mistakenly order industrial gases for this use. Application of the agent to the warts for about 10 seconds as a rapid freeze followed by a slow thaw, and then repeated for 2 to 3 cycles per treatment can hasten resolution of the warts by inducing a local immune response and causing a split within the epidermis (which may result in a blister) to help debulk the wart. Care should be taken to avoid overfreezing, which may result in persistent depigmentation or scarring. Retreatments in the office can be recommended every 2 to 3 weeks to optimize the response, as longer intervals may allow regrowth in between treatments.

For children with numerous warts involving multiple sites, oral cimetidine may be a reasonable option. While randomized controlled trials in adults have not shown cimetidine to be of benefit for treating warts, there is a trend toward improvement in pediatric patients. Smaller clinical trials have indicated a dose-dependent increase in antiviral cytokines as well as a dose-dependent response to clearing warts when using cimetidine. The dosage for oral cimetidine therapy is 25 to 40 mg/kg/day divided tid or 10 mg/kg/dose given tid, with doses not recommended to exceed 2400 mg daily. Side effects may include but are not limited to gastrointestinal upset, diarrhea, and headaches. There is also an increased risk of gynecomastia among adolescent boys using high doses of cimetidine for long periods of time. When employed, a course of 3 months is advised. Because the product in its liquid form is not especially palatable, asking the pharmacist to flavor the product may make the medication more tolerable for young children who cannot take the pill formulation.

Flat Warts

Since these frequently present as multiple lesions, topical salicylic acid preparations as well as destructive modalities are difficult to use with flat warts. Instead, off-label use of imiquimod cream, sinecatechins ointment, and oral cimetidine may be considered either alone or in combination.

In addition, some patients may respond to use of topical retinoids such as tretinoin cream or tazarotene gel. These agents may be applied once nightly for a period of 1 to 3 months in an attempt to accelerate resolution of the warts. It should be noted, however, that these can also induce eczematous skin changes in children with atopic diathesis or sensitive skin. This can be avoided by applying petrolatum around individual lesions before applying the retinoid to the warts.

Children who are amenable to using light cryotherapy may tolerate its use.

Filiform or Digitate Warts

While any of the treatments described previously can be helpful, it is my experience that these warts usually respond best to light cryotherapy with a focus on freezing the base of individual lesions. Resistant lesions may also be amenable to simple curettage or snip excision with appropriate local anesthesia.

Condyloma

Patients with condyloma should be appropriately screened for any history or evidence of sexual abuse.

Given the sensitive location of these lesions, gentler treatment modalities are recommended.

Here, off-label use (based on age, but not indication) of imiquimod cream, sinecatechins ointment, and oral cimetidine may be considered either alone or in combination.

Imiquimod 5% cream is typically applied on Mondays, Wednesdays, and Fridays; left on overnight; and washed off in the morning.

Sinecatechins ointment is typically applied up to 3 times daily; and washed off in the morning. While this agent is usually well-tolerated, some patients may experience irritation, so it may be advisable to start with once-daily application initially, advancing to twice-daily application, and eventually to 3 times daily application over the first couple of weeks so as to avoid excessive irritation.

Whenever using any wart treatments, consistent adherence to home therapeutic regimens, and regular attendance for office treatments provide the best chances for a favorable response to therapy. Also remember that epidermal nevi, which grow in thin lines and are typically present from birth or early childhood, are not warts and so may not respond to therapy as expected (Figure 36-3).

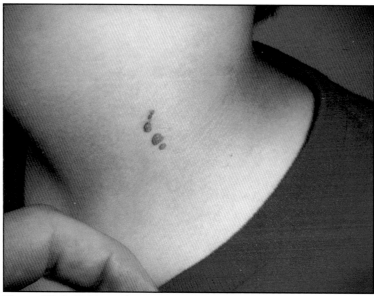

Figure 36-3. Epidermal nevus on the neck, present since birth and recalcitrant to therapy.

Suggested Readings

Fit KE, Williams PC. Use of histamine2-antagonists for the treatment of verruca vulgaris. *Ann Pharmacother.* 2007;41(7):1222-1226. Epub 2007 May 29.

Silverberg NB. Human papillomavirus infections in children. *Curr Opin Pediatr.* 2004;16(4):402-409.

WHAT ARE THE CURRENT RECOMMENDATIONS FOR LYME DISEASE BASED ON THE STAGE AT WHICH THE ILLNESS IS DIAGNOSED?

Brian T. Fisher, DO, MSCE, MPH

Postexposure Management

During the spring, summer, and autumn months, children are often brought to the doctor's office after a tick exposure with questions about whether to pre-emptively treat for Lyme disease. For multiple reasons, I do not advocate prescribing antibiotics to children for this indication. First, even when the tick exposure is known to be an *Ixodes scapularis* or *Ixodes pacificus* tick (the tick species known to harbor *Borrelia burgdorferi* [*B burgdorferi*]), the resultant infection rate is very low. Treating all exposed patients would result in unnecessary antibiotic exposures for a majority of patients. Second, only single-dose doxycycline in adult patients has been evaluated and shown to be somewhat effective in this setting. Amoxicillin has not been evaluated for postexposure management and thus its effectiveness for such is unknown. This then limits the number of children that can receive postexposure prophylaxis. Therefore, most experts agree that for patients with a contraindication for doxycycline it is prudent to monitor for development of an erythema migrans lesion at the site of the original tick bite. Therapy should be initiated should such a rash present.

Early-Localized Lyme Disease

Early-localized disease represents the presence of a single erythema migrans rash located at the site of a recent tick bite. Classically, erythema migrans is an oval erythematous patch with central clearing that is approximately 5 cm in diameter. This rash has the appearance of a "bulls-eye" or "target lesion." Occasionally, the primary erythema migrans patch can present in areas that distort the bulls-eye appearance such as around

Figure 37-1. Atypical appearance of erythema migrans presenting on the dorsum of the left fifth toe.

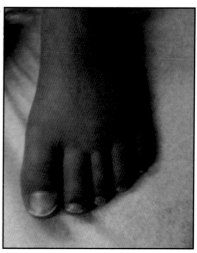

the ear or on the foot (Figure 37-1). In addition to erythema migrans, early-localized disease can be associated with other nonspecific symptoms such as fever, headache, and muscle or joint discomfort. Assuming that the appearance of the rash is consistent with erythema migrans and the patient is from or has recently traveled to a Lyme-endemic region, there is no reason to perform any diagnostic testing as the clinical presentation often precedes the development of antibodies to *B burgdorferi*. Therefore, in the setting of a clinical examination consistent with early-localized disease, it is my practice to initiate doxycycline or amoxicillin therapy. Fourteen days of therapy is appropriate for early-localized disease.

Early-Disseminated and Late-Lyme Disease

In various medical texts and publications, a distinction is often made between early-disseminated and late-Lyme disease. The former typically presents within a few weeks to months of the tick exposure and can be associated with a myriad of clinical presentations including multiple erythema migrans lesions (Figure 37-2), meningitis, cranial nerve palsies, or carditis. Late-Lyme disease often presents as arthritis (most frequently the knee) weeks to months after the initial exposure. In reality, there can be overlap in the timing of onset of each of these presentations and thus defining the clinical entity (eg, meningitis, carditis, or arthritis) is more important in guiding therapeutic decisions then categorizing a patient as early-disseminated or late-Lyme disease. Therefore, the most common clinical presentations and the therapeutic recommendations for each will be discussed. At the time of presentation, a thorough clinical examination should be performed to assess for each of the manifestations mentioned above. Clinical findings should dictate diagnostic and therapeutic interventions. Encephalomyelitis, encephalopathy, and radiculopathy have all been described in relation to Lyme disease. However, these are rare clinical entities for children and thus will not be further discussed here. If the clinician has a concern for these neurologic manifestations, then an infectious disease consult is warranted.

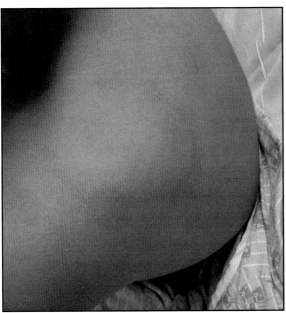

Figure 37-2. One of many large expanding erythematous annular patches on this child with early-disseminated Lyme disease.

Clinical Presentations

EARLY-DISSEMINATED DISEASE WITHOUT OTHER MANIFESTATIONS

When a patient presents with multiple skin lesions consistent with erythema migrans, the diagnosis of Lyme disease should be strongly considered. Assuming that there are no other clinical findings, I will initiate therapy with doxycycline or amoxicillin and send an enzyme immunoassay (EIA) for immunoglobulin M (IgM) and immunoglobulin G (IgG) with reflex if positive to Western immunoblot analysis for confirmation of the infection. At this point in the illness, serologies should be positive but rarely a patient may not have seroconverted. If the clinical presentation is classic for Lyme disease but testing is negative, I will still treat and consider repeating convalescent titers 2 weeks later to confirm the illness. Similar to early-localized disease, 14 days of either doxycycline or amoxicillin is appropriate. Some clinicians elect to treat both early-localized and early-disseminated disease for as long as 21 days but there is no evidence to suggest that longer courses are more effective. In fact, recent data showed that adult patients treated for 10 days with doxycycline had the same outcome as those treated longer.

NEUROLOGIC MANIFESTATIONS OF LYME DISEASE

Neurologic symptoms such as a persistent daily headache, nuchal rigidity, or papilledema on retinal examination should raise the suspicion of Lyme meningitis and result in a lumbar puncture. Analysis of the cerebrospinal fluid (CSF) should focus on the cell count and differential. In my opinion, a patient with positive serologies for Lyme disease and a lymphocytic pleocytosis is enough to establish the diagnosis of Lyme meningitis. Some experts recommend specific CSF Lyme antibody testing and PCR analysis to support the diagnosis of Lyme meningitis. Because the PCR has a poor sensitivity and the CSF antibodies can be difficult to interpret, I do not often order these studies. If a patient has central nervous system (CNS) symptoms, a lymphocytic pleocytosis, and positive Lyme serologies, I will treat for Lyme meningitis. Lyme meningitis should be treated with intravenous (IV) ceftriaxone for 14 days. Some guidelines have suggested longer therapy up to 28 days for CNS disease but this suggestion is not supported by the literature. Thus it has been my practice to limit the duration of treatment to 14 days, as there are inherent risks for continuing therapy (eg, central-line infections, medication toxicities) without defined benefits.

Isolated cranial nerve palsies can also be a clinical presentation of Lyme disease. Most frequently, patients will have a unilateral seventh nerve palsy that results in facial asymmetry on examination. If there are no other neurologic manifestations, then patients with a seventh-nerve palsy do not need to undergo lumbar puncture and can be managed with an oral course of doxycycline or amoxicillin for 14 days. Again, some experts will recommend longer courses for seventh-nerve palsies but limited evidence exists to support these durations. It should be noted that a seventh-nerve palsy often improves on its own over the course of weeks to months regardless of antibiotic administration. The reason for initiating antibiotic therapy in this setting is to reduce the risk of additional Lyme manifestations such as arthritis. Other cranial nerve palsies such as a sixth-nerve palsy or multiple palsies at the same time may be evidence of increased intracranial pressure, and thus additional testing is prudent to evaluate for CNS infection.

LYME CARDITIS

Lyme carditis is relatively rare in children but can manifest as dizziness, dyspnea, or a syncopal episode. Carditis typically is associated with a prolonged PR interval but may result in complete heart block. In patients with suspected carditis, a 12-lead electrocardiogram (EKG) should be performed. I often recommend that patients symptomatic from Lyme carditis be admitted for short-term monitoring even if their heart block is not advanced because the degree of heart block may progress rapidly. Other experts will treat patients without complete heart block in the outpatient setting. Children with complete heart block will likely need temporary pacing and thus admission and consultation with a pediatric cardiologist are necessary. No formal studies have been performed to document the most appropriate antibiotic regimen for Lyme carditis. However, most experts would agree that it is reasonable to administer ceftriaxone intravenously while hospitalized. Once a patient is no longer symptomatic and there is no progression of heart block, I am comfortable transitioning to oral doxycycline or amoxicillin for completion of therapy as an outpatient. A total duration of 14 days is likely adequate but other experts have recommended durations as long as 28 days. It is important to realize that carditis may be the result of an immune-mediated process and not directly related to *B burgdorferi* infection. This is supported by the fact that in certain cases the heart block may persist after completion of a course of antibiotics. In these situations, I do not repeat the course of antibiotics but instead, in consultation with a cardiologist, follow the patient with repeat EKGs to establish resolution.

LYME ARTHRITIS

Lyme arthritis is the primary clinical manifestation associated with late-onset Lyme disease. The knee is the most common joint involved but other large joints (eg, hips, shoulders) and temporomandibular joints can also be affected. The arthritis can present as a monoarticular process but occasionally the arthritis is migratory or involves more than one joint simultaneously. It is important to distinguish the presentation of Lyme arthritis from septic arthritis. Patients often present with a history of joint swelling and mild tenderness to palpation. They are still able to ambulate with some discomfort, which is not typical for patients with a true septic arthritis. Generally, it is not necessary to perform a diagnostic joint aspiration, as the clinical presentation in conjunction with positive serologies is appropriate to make the diagnosis of Lyme arthritis. In some circumstances, the degree of discomfort may be severe enough to warrant evaluation for septic arthritis. A white cell count of less than 50,000 leukocytes/mm^3 is more consistent with Lyme arthritis than septic arthritis. A positive PCR analysis of a joint aspirate sample may also help confirm the diagnosis of Lyme arthritis but is not necessary for diagnosis. Because Lyme arthritis is a late manifestation of the infection, there are often no other clinical symptoms present. By the time a patient develops Lyme arthritis he or she should have mounted an IgG antibody response as measured by EIA and immunoblot techniques. I am often suspicious of a diagnosis of Lyme arthritis in a patient that has only mounted an IgM response and thus I consider other possible diagnoses (eg, septic arthritis, rheumatologic condition, or an oncologic process).

Reasonable pediatric data exist to support an oral course of either doxycycline or amoxicillin for the treatment of Lyme arthritis assuming no other symptoms (ie, CNS manifestations) are present. The duration of therapy for Lyme arthritis is less well established and often a range of 14 to 28 days is recommended. In my practice, I prescribe 28 days of therapy but expect that future studies will reveal that shorter courses are effective as well. The swelling associated with Lyme arthritis may persist or recur after completion of an antibiotic course. If the swelling persists for a number of weeks off antibiotics or if the swelling improves but recurs weeks later, I will often recommend a second course of antibiotics. Some experts recommend that when a second course is prescribed it should be IV ceftriaxone. There are no data to support the superiority of IV ceftriaxone as compared to a repeat course of oral antibiotics. If there was no clinical improvement after the first course of oral therapy and adherence can be confirmed, then I will consider administering a 2-week course of ceftriaxone. Otherwise, I often recommend a repeat course of oral antibiotics because of the inherent risks of prolonged IV therapy without a clear benefit. Finally, some patients will persist with arthritis even after a second course of antibiotics. For these patients, the persistent swelling may well be secondary to an autoimmune process and thus I consult with a pediatric rheumatologist for recommendations of anti-inflammatory therapies.

Treatment Options

Antibiotic regimen guidelines for each of the aforementioned presentations are detailed in Table 37-1. Doxycycline should be reserved for children 8 years of age or older. Patients prescribed doxycycline should be warned of the risk of photosensitivity, nausea, headaches, and to avoid taking the medication with calcium-containing foods, which can inhibit absorption. Cefuroxime is an oral alternative to doxycycline or amoxicillin while cefotaxime and penicillin are IV alternatives to ceftriaxone.

Table 37-1

Suggested Antibiotic Regimens by Clinical Presentation of Lyme Disease

Clinical Presentation	Medication	Route	Pediatric Dose	Duration
Single or multiple erythema migrans lesion(s)	Doxycycline* OR Amoxicillin	Oral Oral	4 mg/kg/d (max 200 mg/d) divided twice a day 50 mg/kg/d (max 1.5 g/d) divided 3 times a day	14 to 21 days
Isolated facial nerve palsy	Doxycycline* OR Amoxicillin	Oral Oral	4 mg/kg/d (max 200 mg/d) divided twice a day 50 mg/kg/d (max 1.5 g/d) divided 3 times a day	14 to 21 days
Meningitis	Ceftriaxone	IV	75 to 100 mg/kg/d (up to 2 g) once a day	14 to 28 days
Carditis Inpatient Outpatient	Ceftriaxone Doxycycline* OR Amoxicillin	IV Oral Oral	75 to 100 mg/kg/d (up to 2 g) once a day 4 mg/kg/d (max 200 mg/d) divided twice a day 50 mg/kg/d (max 1.5 g/d) divided 3 times a day	Until discharge To complete 14 to 21 days total
Arthritis	Doxycycline* OR Amoxicillin	Oral Oral	4 mg/kg/d (max 200 mg/d) divided twice a day 50 mg/kg/d (max 1.5 g/d) divided 3 times a day	28 days

IV indicates intravenous

*Doxycycline should be avoided in children less than 8 years of age.

Suggested Readings

Halperin JJ, Shapiro ED, Logigian E, et al. Practice parameter: treatment of nervous system Lyme disease (an evidence-based review): report of the Quality Standards Subcommittee of the American Academy of Neurology. *Neurology.* 2007;69(1):91-102.

Kowalski TJ, Tata S, Berth W, Mathiason MA, Agger WA. Antibiotic treatment duration and long-term outcomes of patients with early lyme disease from a lyme disease-hyperendemic area. *Clin Infect Dis.* 2010;50(4):512-520.

Murray TS, Shapiro ED. Lyme disease. *Clin Lab Med.* 2010;30(1):311-328.

Wormser GP, Dattwyler RJ, Shapiro ED, et al. The clinical assessment, treatment, and prevention of lyme disease, human granulocytic anaplasmosis, and babesiosis: clinical practice guidelines by the Infectious Diseases Society of America. *Clin Infect Dis.* 2006;43(9):1089-1134. Epub 2006 Oct 2.

WHAT GENITAL LESIONS SHOULD MAKE ME SUSPECT CHILD ABUSE?

Maj. Sarah M. Frioux, MD and Joanne Wood, MD, MSHP

You should consider the possibility of sexual abuse when evaluating a child with a traumatic or infectious genital lesion. As will be discussed, certain lesions are highly specific for sexual abuse while others may be nonspecific or more consistent with a medical disorder or accidental injury. It is important to remember that the vast majority of children disclosing sexual abuse do not have physical evidence of injury or infection on examination. Sexual abuse describes involvement of children and adolescents in developmentally inappropriate sexual activities to which they are unable to consent and which they cannot comprehend. Violent assault causing severe injuries is the exception in child sexual abuse, as sexual abusers often exploit the power differential between victim and perpetrator to manipulate children into complying with sexual activity.

Your role as a mandated reporter requires you to report reasonable suspicions of inappropriate sexual contact. The standards for mandatory reporting vary from state to state. Therefore, it is important that you acquaint yourself with the laws of the state in which you practice. Referral to or consultation with a child abuse specialist may be appropriate to assist with the evaluation, diagnosis, and treatment of suspected sexual abuse.

Traumatic Injuries

ACUTE TRAUMA

Acute lacerations or ecchymoses of the hymen or anus are consistent with recent blunt force penetrating trauma to the genital or anal area and should raise a high level of concern for sexual abuse.[1] Other acute genital injuries such as bruising or lacerations of the vulva, penis, scrotum, perineum, or perianal area may be caused by sexual abuse or physical abuse but may also result from nonpenetrating accidental injury. Such findings should be accompanied by a clear and plausible description of the accident.

Remote Trauma

Injuries to the hymen often fully heal; however, some children may have residual findings especially in cases in which a laceration transects the hymen by extending from the rim to the base. Healed hymenal transections and missing areas of hymen in the posterior half of the hymen are highly suggestive of prior penetrating trauma and should raise concern for sexual abuse, even in the absence of a disclosure of abuse. Findings such as deep notches in the posterior hymen may be consistent with healed traumatic injury, but may also represent normal variants in genital anatomy. Scarring of the posterior four-chette or anus may be consistent with healed traumatic injury, but must be distinguished from normal variants such as diastasis ani and midline fusion defects.

Sexually Transmitted Infections

Human Papillomaviruses

Human papillomavirus (HPV) infection frequently produces warts, which are benign epithelial proliferations. Anogenital infection may produce large, skin-colored lesions known as condyloma accuminatum. In adults, anogenital HPV is primarily sexually transmitted. However, emerging evidence indicates that sexual transmission is not the only route of transmission in young children.[2] HPV can be spread by vertical transmission, even from a mother without a history of genital warts or abnormal Pap smears, because many adults with HPV infection are asymptomatic and most infections are transient. In addition, children may be inoculated with HPV by a caregiver innocently during toileting assistance and diaper changes or because of poor hand hygiene. Children may also self-inoculate with HPV.

When evaluating children presenting with anogenital condyloma accuminatum, the caregiver should be asked about a maternal history of HPV infection, presence of warts in caregivers, and any concerns for sexual abuse. Verbal children should be separated from their caregiver and asked about a history of inappropriate sexual contact using nonleading questions. A physical examination including genital examination and testing for other sexually transmitted infections (STIs) should also be performed. If genital injuries or coinfection with another STI is identified, a high level of concern for sexual abuse should be raised. However, the presence of HPV infection itself is not diagnostic of sexual abuse.

Herpes Simplex Viruses

Genital herpes infection begins as a painful, vesicular eruption and progresses to characteristic ulcerative lesions. Herpes simplex virus (HSV) is transmitted through direct contact with infected secretions and has an incubation period of 2 days to 2 weeks.[3] While HSV-1 and HSV-2 are classically associated with oral and genital infections, respectively, there is significant crossover of presentation, so that HSV type is no longer strongly associated with site of infection in some geographic areas. In addition, genital HSV lesions can arise from autoinoculation from oral herpes lesions, making determination of primary versus secondary infection critical in understanding the origin of the infection.

As with HPV infection, children with genital HSV should undergo a history, physical examination including genital examination, and testing for other STIs. Genital HSV infection in children is highly concerning for sexual abuse. In the absence of a history of autoinoculation from a nongenital HSV infection, cases of genital HSV should be reported to child protective services.

CHANCRES

Primary syphilis lesions present as painless, indurated ulcers at the site of primary inoculation. Chancres typically appear about 3 weeks after exposure, and resolve spontaneously within a few weeks. As this dermatologic manifestation of syphilis is specific to transmission outside the neonatal period, any child presenting with a chancre should be reported to child protective services, even without disclosure of sexual abuse by the child.[4]

OTHER SEXUALLY TRANSMITTED INFECTIONS

Chlamydia trachomatis is the infectious agent responsible for lymphogranuloma venereum, which presents initially as a painful genital ulcer and unilateral, painful lymphadenopathy. This presentation is uncommon in children but has been reported.[5] *Haemophilus ducreyi* infection presents with an erythematous, tender papule and progresses to a necrotic, ulcerated lesion, which may ultimately resolve spontaneously. This lesion is often associated with unilateral inguinal lymphadenitis. There is no known route of nonsexual transmission for *H ducreyi*.[6] Children with *C trachomatis* or *H ducreyi* infections should be evaluated for sexual abuse, including screening for other STIs and referred to child protective services.

INFECTIONS NOT CONCERNING FOR ABUSE

Several non-STIs can present with genital lesions but are not concerning for sexual abuse. Molluscum contagiosum lesions can appear in the genital area and are distinguished from condyloma accuminatum by their distinctive smooth texture and central umbilication. Perineal group A streptococcal infection is characterized by erythematous, painful vaginal, or perianal mucosa and can be confirmed by routine genital culture. Other nonsexually transmitted causes of vulvovaginitis can also be detected by genital culture, including *Candida* and Group A *Streptococcus*. In addition, some children with systemic viral infections, such as Epstein-Barr virus, can present with exquisitely painful, hemorrhagic, Lipschütz ulcerations of the labia and vagina. Pediculosis pubis and scabies may be transmitted from nonsexual contact and should not be considered indicative of sexual abuse.

Differential Diagnosis of Genital Lesions

A number of other noninfectious childhood diseases can present with genital lesions that are not concerning for child sexual abuse.[7] Labial lichen sclerosus et atrophicus presents with pink, ivory, or white atrophic areas of skin with wrinkling and increased fragility. Minor injuries to the atrophic skin may produce hemorrhagic, vesicular, or bullous lesions. Genital ulcers can occur with autoimmune conditions, systemic illnesses, and drug reactions.

Labial adhesions are common in preschool children and occur when labial skin becomes inflamed and irritated, and labial edges adhere. The degree of involvement of the labia is variable; some children have a very small posterior segment of labial adhesion while others present with only a small opening through which urine can exit. Urethral prolapse is also seen most commonly in young children and appears as a doughnut-shaped mass completely surrounding the urethra. The exposed urethral skin may become ulcerated or necrotic due to friction against the child's skin or clothing and may bleed. Both severe labial adhesions and urethral prolapse can be treated with topical estrogen cream if symptoms are significant.

Summary

While children may occasionally present with genital injuries or infections that are concerning for child sexual abuse, it is important to remember that the vast majority of sexually abused children have no injuries or symptoms from their abuse. In addition, a number of genital findings are associated with medical conditions and are not due to abuse. A diagnosis of child sexual abuse requires careful consideration of the child's history, physical examination, and laboratory evaluation. Any reasonable suspicion of child abuse should be reported to the child's local child protective services agency.

References

1. Adams JA. Guidelines for medical care of children evaluated for suspected sexual abuse: an update for 2008. *Curr Opin Obstet Gynecol.* 2008;20(5):435-441.
2. Sinclair KA, Woods CR, Kirse DJ, Sinal SH. Anogenital and respiratory tract human papillomavirus infections among children: age, gender, and potential transmission through sexual abuse. *Pediatrics.* 2005;116(4):815-825.
3. American Academy of Pediatrics. Herpes Simplex. In: Pickering LK, Baker CJ, Kimberlin DW, Long SS, eds. *Red Book: 2009 Report of the Committee on Infectious Diseases.* 28th ed. Elk Grove Village, IL: American Academy of Pediatrics; 2009:363-373.
4. Christian CW, Lavelle J, Bell LM. Preschoolers with syphilis. *Pediatrics.* 1999;103(1):E4.
5. Darville T. *Chlamydia trachomatis* infections in neonates and young children. *Semin Pediatr Infect Dis.* 2005;16(4):235-244.
6. American Academy of Pediatrics. Chancroid. In: Pickering LK, Baker CJ, Kimberlin DW, Long SS, eds. *Red Book: 2009 Report of the Committee on Infectious Diseases.* 28th ed. Elk Grove Village, IL: American Academy of Pediatrics; 2009:250-252.
7. Kellogg ND, Parra JM, Menard S. Children with anogenital symptoms and signs referred for sexual abuse evaluations. *Arch Pediatr Adolesc Med.* 1998;152(7):634-641.

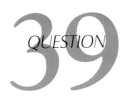

HOW SHOULD I APPROACH GENITAL ULCERS IN SEXUALLY ACTIVE TEENS?

Maj. Sarah M. Frioux, MD and Joanne Wood, MD, MSHP

While the diagnosis and treatment of most genital ulcerations is not complex, the presence of this finding in an adolescent patient raises a unique set of concerns. We will discuss the diagnosis of genital ulcerations in this age group as well as the considerations that are specific to this particular population. Although not all genital ulcers are caused by sexually transmitted infections (STIs), herpes simplex virus (HSV) and syphilis are the most common cause of genital ulcers in young sexually active patients. When presented with an adolescent patient with genital ulcers, evaluation for HSV and syphilis must be performed. In areas of high prevalence, testing for *Haemophilus ducreyi* should be performed. Based on the clinical presentation and local epidemiology, testing for less common STI causes of genital ulcers including donovanosis should be considered. Nonvenereal causes of genital ulcers should also be considered and evaluated for, especially if STI testing is negative.

Sexually Transmitted Genital Ulcers

HERPES SIMPLEX VIRUS

Genital herpes infection is often the first infection that clinicians associate with painful genital ulcers. The characteristic course of primary herpes begins as a painful eruption of groups of vesicles, which progress to ulcerations, and ultimately resolve spontaneously.[1] Infection with HSV is lifelong, as the virus remains latent in the sensory ganglia until reactivation. Recurrent HSV eruptions may have a prodrome of itching, followed by onset of characteristic herpes lesions. Despite the clear presentation of many patients with HSV, some individuals remain asymptomatic during primary and reactivated infection. In spite of the lack of obvious herpes lesions, these asymptomatic individuals shed virus and can infect others, making it difficult to identify the source of infection for some patients. HSV can be confirmed through viral culture or polymerase chain reaction of skin lesions. Antiviral therapy is indicated for primary and recurrent HSV infection, and may lessen symptoms and shorten the duration of illness. Suppressive therapy to reduce the frequency of recurrences should also be offered to patients.

SYPHILIS

Chancres are the painless, indurated ulcers that appear during the primary stage of syphilis.[2] They typically appear at the site of primary inoculation about 3 weeks after exposure and resolve spontaneously within a few weeks. A definitive diagnosis of syphilis is made when *Treponema pallidum* spirochetes are seen on microscopic darkfield examination or direct fluorescent antibody testing of secretions is positive. Nontreponemal serologic testing (eg, rapid plasma reagin or Venereal Disease Research Laboratory) is not specific for *T pallidum* but is abnormal during active syphilis infections. Fluorescent treponemal antibody absorption is a specific treponemal serologic test, but it is known to remain positive long after the infection has been treated. By considering treponemal and nontreponemal serologies together, presumptive diagnosis of syphilis is possible. The course of treatment for syphilis is dependent on the stage of disease and presenting symptoms.

CHANCROID

H ducreyi infection initially presents with an erythematous, tender papule that develops into a superficial, painful, nonindurated ulcer.[3] Chancroid lesions may present in multiples or as single lesions and can be associated with unilateral inguinal lymphadenitis and bubo formation. These lesions often self-resolve over a period of weeks. Males may also present with a purulent urethritis. There is a high rate of coinfection with other STIs, and the presence of chancroid lesions increases the risk of human immunodeficiency virus (HIV) transmission. This infection is also highly associated with prostitution and use of illicit drugs. Definitive diagnosis of *H ducreyi* infection, which is rare in the United States and Europe, is made by culture of the lesion. However, culture for *H ducreyi* may not be available and is not very sensitive. Thus a probable clinical diagnosis of chancroid can be made in patients with more than one painful ulcer if the clinical presentation and appearance of lesions and lymphadenopathy are typical of chancroid, and testing for HSV and *T pallidum* is negative.[4]

LYMPHOGRANULOMA VENEREUM

Lymphogranuloma venereum (LGV) is an invasive lymphatic infection caused by specific serologic variants (serovars) of *Chlamydia trachomatis* (*C trachomatis*).[5] LGV lesions begin as painless genital ulcers that may be unnoticed by the patient. Within a few weeks, unilateral painful lymphadenopathy develops. Anal infection with LGV serovars can result in severe proctocolitis due to direct exposure of the rectal mucosa. Diagnosis of *C trachomatis* infection is achieved either through culture or nucleic acid amplification testing. While culture remains the gold standard, the obligate intracellular nature of *Chlamydia* species requires that all culture specimens include adequate epithelial cells. This can be technically difficult to achieve, decreasing the sensitivity of the culture. Nucleic acid amplification testing is more sensitive than culture but is commercially available only for urethral and vaginal samples.

GRANULOMA INGUINALE (DONOVANOSIS)

Infection with *Klebsiella granulomatis* is endemic in certain tropical regions.[6] It presents as a pruritic papule at the site of primary transmission, which later ulcerates and spreads through skin-to-skin contact along skin folds. Ulcers are relatively painless but friable, and prone to easy bleeding. Lymph node involvement is infrequent. Diagnosis is made by biopsy and smear preparation, which demonstrates characteristic Donovan bodies.

Special Considerations in Evaluating and Treating Adolescents With Sexually Transmitted Infections

PRIVACY, CONFIDENTIALLY, AND CONSENT

All adolescent patients should be offered the option to discuss their concerns alone with their physician. A history of present illness obtained in front of a parent may differ significantly from what might be shared privately between the doctor and patient. It is often most effective if the physician asks the parent to leave as a matter of course, without asking the patient if he or she desires his or her parent to leave. If the patient objects, then the parent may stay; if the patient desires the parent to leave, then he or she is not put in the position of explaining this to his or her parent, who may not understand the purpose of this procedure. The history should focus on the present illness as well as past medical history and sexual history. The adolescent should be asked about family or dating violence as well, since adolescents are at increased risk for sexual abuse compared to younger children.

Examinations should always be performed with a chaperone, regardless of the gender of the patient or provider. This chaperone could be a parent but is preferably a trained member of the medical staff who can assist in examination procedures and serve as an unbiased witness to the examination. Treatment decisions should be discussed directly with the patient regardless of age.

Laws regarding the privacy concerns and health decision-making rights of adolescents vary from state to state and it is important for you to acquaint yourself with the laws of the state in which you practice. However, minors may consent for their own health services for STIs in all 50 states and the District of Columbia and parental notification for STI services is not required, except in a few limited circumstances.

SEXUALLY TRANSMITTED INFECTION SCREENING

You should screen adolescents with STI-related ulcers for other STIs due to the high rate of coinfection.

Testing for *Neisseria gonorrhoeae, C trachomatis,* and HIV should be performed. Patients presenting within 72 hours of unprotected sexual contact may benefit from STI prophylaxis, as well as HIV postexposure prophylaxis. Pregnancy testing should also be considered in female patients with evidence of an STI.

Role As a Mandated Reporter

In addition to providing treatment for the STI, you must also consider whether the adolescent acquired the STI through consensual intercourse and was legally able to consent. Even if the adolescent assented to the encounter, sexual contact between an adult and adolescent patient is illegal if it violates age-of-consent laws. Laws dictating the age at which adolescents may legally consent to sexual activity vary from state to state. Therefore, it is important that you are familiar with your local laws. Your role as a mandated reporter requires you to report any reasonable suspicions of inappropriate sexual contact.[4]

Nonsexually Transmitted Genital Ulcers

Although STIs are the most common cause of genital ulcers in sexually active adolescents, ulcers can also result from non-STIs and from noninfectious causes. Systemic viral infections, including Epstein-Barr virus and HIV, and autoimmune conditions, such as inflammatory bowel disease and Behçet disease, can present with exquisitely painful, hemorrhagic ulcerations of the labia and vagina. A thorough review of systems including history of recent upper respiratory symptoms, diarrhea, abdominal pain, oral ulcers, blood clots, visual symptoms, pyoderma gangrenosum as well as a thorough family history can help guide work-up in noninfectious causes of ulceration. Fixed drug eruption, trauma, psoriasis, malignancy, and excoriation of nonulcerative lesions can also lead to genital ulcers. Biopsy may be considered for unusual or chronic lesions of unclear etiology that do not respond to therapy.

References

1. American Academy of Pediatrics. Herpes Simplex. In: Pickering L, Baker C, Kimberlin D, Long S, eds. *Red Book: 2009 Report of the Committee on Infectious Diseases*. 28th ed. Elk Grove Village, IL: American Academy of Pediatrics; 2009:363-373.
2. Kent ME, Romanelli F. Reexamining syphilis: an update on epidemiology, clinical manifestations, and management. *Ann Pharmacother*. 2008;42(2):226-236.
3. American Academy of Pediatrics. Chancroid. In: Pickering L, Baker C, Kimberlin D, Long S, eds. *Red Book: 2009 Report of the Committee on Infectious Diseases*. 28th ed. Elk Grove Village, IL: American Academy of Pediatrics; 2009:250-252.
4. Workowski KA, Berman S. Sexually transmitted diseases treatment guidelines, 2010. *MMWR Recomm Rep*. 2010;59(RR-12):1-110.
5. White JA. Manifestations and management of lymphogranuloma venereum. *Curr Opin Infect Dis*. 2009; 22(1):57-66.
6. Richens J. The diagnosis and treatment of donovanosis (granuloma inguinale). *Genitourin Med*. 1991;67(6): 441-452.

SECTION VI

PIGMENTARY AND HAIR DISORDERS

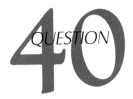

WHAT WORK-UP SHOULD BE DONE FOR PATIENTS WITH VITILIGO?

Leslie Castelo-Soccio, MD, PhD

Vitiligo is a disorder of acquired depigmentation of skin and mucous membranes. It is a multifactorial polygenic disorder that is likely related to genetic and environmental factors. It is most commonly considered an autoimmune disease with alteration in humoral and cellular immunity leading to destruction of melanocytes in the epidermis. Other autoimmune diseases including Graves disease and Hashimoto thyroiditis as well as alopecia areata and pernicious anemia have been associated with vitiligo. Oxidative stress has also been proposed to play an essential role in vitiligo. There are a few studies that suggest that accumulation of free radicals toxic to melanocytes lead to their destruction. While vitiligo is seen in childhood, the average age of onset is 20 years old. Vitiligo occurs with a prevalence of 0.5% to 1%. Most typically, it is a chronic persistent disease with periods of relative inactivity (remission) and shorter periods when depigmentation occurs. Spontaneous repigmentation can occur and is more common in segmental or focal vitiligo.

Vitiligo can be classified as localized or generalized. Localized vitiligo includes segmental, focal, and mucosal variants and is more common in children. Focal vitiligo is characterized by one or more patches in one area, most commonly in the distribution of the trigeminal nerve. Segmental vitiligo similarly refers to one or more patches in a dermatomal or quasidermatomal pattern. More than half of patients with segmental vitiligo have patches of white hair or poliosis. This type of vitiligo is not associated with thyroid or other autoimmune disorders. Mucosal vitiligo occurs when only mucous membranes are affected. Generalized vitiligo can be divided into acrofacial where depigmentation occurs on the distal fingers and periorificial areas, vulgaris where the patches are scattered widely, and mixed where multiple types of vitiligo occur in combination. Universal vitiligo is the least common and occurs with complete or near-complete depigmentation. It is often associated with multiple endocrinopathy syndrome.

Diagnosing vitiligo is the first step of management. In its classic form, it is easily recognized and diagnosed. Symmetrical depigmented areas are identified or focal areas/segmental areas of depigmentation are identified (Figure 40-1). White patches in the scalp

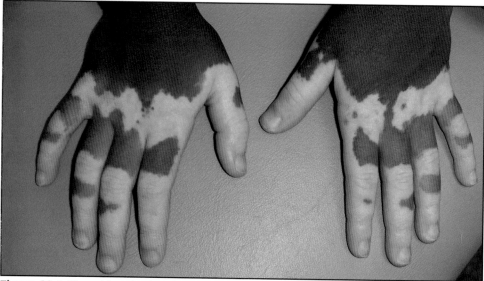

Figure 40-1. Dorsal hands showing symmetric bilateral depigmentation accentuated over frictional areas.

with white hairs are also another presentation. Genital areas are often involved in vitiligo. Vitiligo can also start with a white circular patch around a "halo" nevus when the body is attacking the nevus because it has the most abundant collection of melanocytes. Halo nevi can be the hallmark of impending vitiligo but not all patients with halo nevi will develop vitiligo. Depigmentation of the hands, face, and more visible areas of the body can be psychologically difficult, and part of the treatment includes evaluation of impact on quality of life and self-esteem.

It is important to distinguish vitiligo from other hypopigmented disorders, including pityriasis alba, tinea versicolor, nevus anemicus, or ash leaf macules seen in tuberous sclerosis. In general, hypopigmented skin will not highlight nearly as impressively with a Wood lamp as the depigmented skin of vitiligo. Pityriasis alba is a hypopigmentation typically on the cheeks of children with atopic dermatitis, which again will not highlight extensively with a Wood lamp. Nevus anemicus is a congenital vascular anomaly that presents clinically as a hypopigmented macule or patch. The lesion is white appearing due to a localized hypersensitivity to catecholamines with resultant vasoconstriction. In tuberous sclerosis, patients can present with hypopigmented macules. Again, these can be distinguished from vitiligo by Wood lamp examination. Vitiligo should also be distinguished from genetic disorders characterized by localized lack of pigment including Waardenberg and piebaldism. Waardenberg is associated with a white forelock, broad nasal root, and hypopigmented irides. Piebaldism is distinguished by a white forelock and white patches in the central chest and extremities present since birth in a symmetric distribution. Additionally, dyspigmentation from chronic inflammatory disease can also be mistaken for vitiligo. This postinflammatory hypopigmentation is most common in atopic dermatitis or in patients with a history of other inflammatory skin diseases. Rarely malignancy can mimic vitiligo. Mycosis fungoides is a type of cutaneous lymphoma that can present as hypopigmented patches. Vitiligo-like depigmentation can occur in patients with malignant melanoma. The sites may be remote from the original melanoma but this is very rare in childhood.

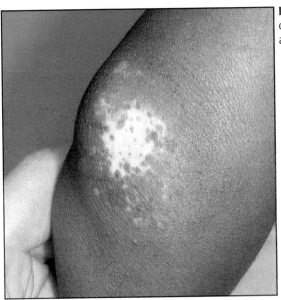

Figure 40-2. Extensor knee showing islands of repigmentation after topical steroid therapy.

Although diagnosis of vitiligo is typically made on the basis of clinical findings and use of a black light, occasionally a biopsy can help distinguish vitiligo from other hypopigmented disorders. Since patients with vitiligo have a slightly higher propensity to develop autoimmune thyroid disease or other autoimmune diseases, clinicians and patients should be aware of the signs and symptoms that suggest the onset of hypothyroidism, diabetes, or other autoimmune diseases. In one study, a history of autoimmune disease in a family member was obtained in approximately 32% of adult patients with vitiligo. Adult prevalence of thyroid disease in patients with vitiligo is 5% and should thus be tested for thyroid dysfunction.

Routine testing for thyroid dysfunction is not necessary in children unless a thorough review of systems suggests growth abnormalities, heat or cold intolerance, weight gain, unusual fatigue, constipation, or changes in bowel habits. Appropriate testing should be obtained if signs and symptoms develop. Thyroid autoantibodies and thyroid-stimulating hormone can be used to screen for thyroid disease. A complete blood count can help rule out anemia and a fasting glucose can help screen for diabetes.

Topical steroids (potency dependent on age of the patient) and topical calcineurin inhibitors are the mainstay of topical therapy. In most children between the ages of 2 and 10, class 4 or 5 steroids are a good place to start therapy. Topical pimecrolimus or tacrolimus has a better side effect profile than high-potency topical steroids and should be considered as steroid-sparing agents, although parents should be made aware of the black box warning about risk of lymphoma. Ultraviolet B (UVB) light is also effective therapy although it can be time intensive, requiring two to three sessions of light therapy a week for 6 to 12 weeks on average. Localized UVB therapy with excimer light can also be used. This provides the benefit of not treating large portions of normal skin with UVB. When vitiligo repigments, it typically starts with small islands of repigmentation, which then expand slowly (Figure 40-2). Active nonintervention can also be considered and is often the most reasonable option. Clinicians should also assess psychological and quality-of-life effects. Psychological counseling should be offered to children and their parents if they are distraught over the disease.

Suggested Readings

Counts D, Varma SK. Hypothyroidism in children. *Pediatr Rev.* 2009;30(7):251-258.

Gawkrodger DJ, Ormerrod AD, Shaw L. Guideline for the diagnosis and management of vitiligo. *Br J Dermatol.* 2008; 159(5):1051-1076.

Gawkrodger DJ, Ormerod AD, Shaw L, et al. Concise evidence based guideline on diagnosis and management. *Postgrad Med J.* 2010;86(1018):466-471.

Mattoo SK, Handa S, Kaur L. Psychiatric morbididty in vitiligo: prevalence correlates in India. *J Eur Acad Dermatol Venerol.* 2002;16(6):573-578.

Papadopoulos L, Bor R, Legg C. Coping with the disfiguring effects of vitiligo: a preliminary investigation into the effects of cognitive-behavioural therapy. *Br J Med Psychol.* 1999;72(Pt 3):385-396.

Westerhof W, Nieuweboer-Krobotova L. Treatment of vitiligo with UV-B radiation versus topical psoralen plus UV-A. *Arch Dermatol.* 1997;133(12):1525-1528.

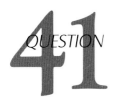

WHAT WORK-UP SHOULD BE DONE FOR PATIENTS WITH ALOPECIA?

Leslie Castelo-Soccio, MD, PhD

There are four common types of hair loss in children: alopecia related to tinea capitis, alopecia areata, traction alopecia, and telogen effluvium. Of course hair loss is not limited to these categories. Trichotillosis (formerly trichotillomania), a compulsion to pull out hair consciously or unconsciously, may also produce alopecia (see Question 45). Rarer reasons for acquired alopecia in children include pressure-induced alopecia that can be seen after prolonged surgery, alopecia related to nutritional deficiency or toxic ingestion, and androgenetic alopecia (male or female pattern baldness). Temporal triangular alopecia, aplasia cutis, and nevus sebaceus should be considered in congenital alopecia.

Work-up is dependent on the type of alopecia. The first step is to determine the cause of the hair loss. Clues to the type of hair loss include evidence of scale, hair breakage, location of the hair loss, age of the child, and whether there are other comorbidities.

One approach is to start by evaluating for scale, alopecia, and occipital lymphadenopathy. If present, alopecia is caused by tinea capitis until proven otherwise. Tinea capitis is a disease caused by fungal infection of the scalp, with a propensity for attacking hair shafts and follicles. It is also called "ringworm of the scalp." The fungus lives in or on the hair shaft and causes the hairs to break. In Figure 41-1, there are areas of "black dot" tinea on the right and areas of alopecia areata demonstrated by completely bald skin on the left and nuchal areas. The patch of hair loss is often round and the scalp can take on a black-dotted stubble appearance from hair shafts broken off at the surface. There may also be itching. The condition is transmitted by contact from one infected child to another through the sharing of combs, brushes, hats, barrettes, pillows, and bath towels or from an infected animal to a human. Small breaks in the scalp such as those from close cutting of the hair provide entry for the microscopic fungus. Children 3 to 10 years of age are more susceptible and boys more so than girls. Without treatment, the hair loss can be considerable, and some children will develop a boggy, tender inflammatory swelling of the scalp known as a kerion. If tinea capitis is suspected, a dermatophyte screen (fungal culture specific for dermatophytes) should be performed. This can easily be done by brushing

Figure 41-1. Areas of "black dot" tinea on the right and areas of alopecia areata demonstrated by completely bald skin on the left and nuchal areas.

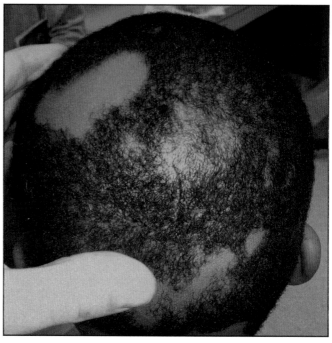

the affected scalp with a new sterile toothbrush or bacterial swab, which is then sent to a microbiology laboratory for culture and evaluation. Families should be instructed to use topical antifungal shampoos and creams until dermatophyte screen results are available. Hairbrushes, combs, and hats should be washed in hot water. If the dermatophyte screen is positive, oral and topical antifungals are recommended for treatment.

The most commonly used oral antifungal in the United States for tinea capitis is griseofulvin microsized. It is typically taken for 4 to 6 weeks at a dose of 10 to 20 mg/kg/day in children over 2 years of age. More extended off-label 6- to 8-week therapy at 20 mg/kg/day is often thought to be more effective and still well tolerated. It is critical that it is taken with a fatty meal to maximize its absorption. Selenium sulfide shampoo, used twice a week, has been shown to shorten the course of tinea capitis. Topical antifungal creams alone usually do not help in killing the fungus unless children are under 1 year of age and their hair is fine. Shaving the hair or giving the child a close haircut is unnecessary. Even though the infection is still visible, a child with tinea capitis may return to school after oral medication is started and the scalp receives at least one washing with shampoo. Alternatives to griseofulvin include terbinafine, which can be orally dosed in children over 4 years. Typical dosing is for 6 weeks at 62.5 mg daily for children under 20 kg, 125 mg daily for children 20 to 40 kg, and 250 mg daily for children over 40 kg. These can be sprinkled on food or in a drink. It is uncommon for dermatophyte infections of the scalp to be resistant to both of these therapies.

If dermatophyte screen is negative but there is still scaling, especially in preadolescent children, atopic dermatitis is a commonly overlooked cause of alopecia. Treatment should include midpotency topical steroids to the scalp to decrease scale and itch. Chronic rubbing can produce a look of alopecia. Extensive seborrheic dermatitis or sebopsoriasis in the scalp can also cause hair loss but the more prominent clinical feature is scaling

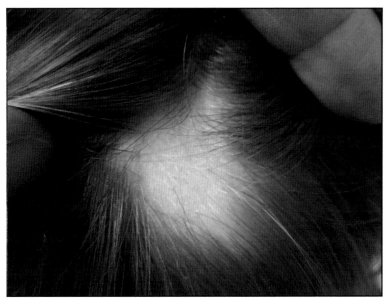

Figure 41-2. Alopecic nonscaley area regrowing with lighter hairs in alopecia areata.

and erythema. This typically can be identified by greasy scale in the scalp particularly along hairlines and is also found along the ears, eyebrows, and around the nasal ala. Low-potency topical steroids such as fluocinolone 0.01% solution in combination with antidandruff shampoos can be effective to improve seborrheic dermatitis and growth of hair in the scalp and topical antifungals such as ketoconazole 2% cream can be effective on the face.

If there is no scale and there are patches of smooth, soft, sometimes pink, scalp, which looks like normal hairless skin in round or oval shapes, hair loss is likely alopecia areata (see upper left and nuchal areas of Figure 41-1). The most typical history is sudden appearance of circular, completely bald patches in the scalp. The hair at the borders of these patches is loose. Eyebrows, eyelashes, and body hair should be evaluated for hair loss because hair loss can be universal. Nails should be evaluated for characteristic nail pits (small indentations in the nails) that are often present. Regrown hairs can look tapered at the ends and are known as exclamation point hairs and will be smaller in caliber and lighter or white in color (Figure 41-2). A smaller number of children develop what is known as an ophiasis pattern of hair loss, which is hair loss in a band on the posterior scalp that extends anteriorly to the parietal scalp above the ears. Fortunately, we can advise parents that the majority of children with alopecia areata are otherwise completely healthy and that their hair loss is not contagious. While stress has been implicated as one factor that contributes to alopecia areata, there is no evidence that psychological stress/nervousness contributes to this disorder. In 20% of cases, there is another family member with a history of alopecia areata.

It is not necessary to perform blood work on these patients if their review of systems does not suggest thyroid dysfunction, diabetes, or other autoimmune phenomenon. Some advocate checking zinc and iron levels and supplementing if either are low to provide an optimal environment for hair growth. Fortunately, over 80% of children will regrow hair over the following 12 months. In my experience, the longer a child goes without hair growth in a particular area, the less likely that it will grow back.

If hair loss is only on the sides or in the front of the scalp in a female child, consider traction alopecia. Traction alopecia is physical damage to the hair by putting constant pressure on the hair, which results in pulling hair out from the roots. Constant harsh styling, including teasing, combing, washing, and blow drying as well as hot combings, straightening, and coloring, can make hair more fragile and more likely to break. Styles that apply tension to the hair, such as tight ponytails and tight braiding, can also damage the hair. Recommended treatment for children's traction alopecia is to handle the hair gently, as little as possible, and use looser hairstyles. A general rule is to make sure a finger can be inserted in between the hair and the scalp to assure the hair is not pulled too tightly when braided or put into a ponytail. The hair will usually return, but regrowth can be slow. Injured hair follicles do not heal quickly and often take 3 or more months before they are back to their growing phase.

Trichotillosis is another cause of trauma to the hair (see Question 45). It is caused by the habit of twirling or plucking the hair. It is thought to be an obsessive-compulsive disorder that can be extremely difficult to treat since the patient usually feels compelled to pluck his or her hair. The hair loss is patchy and characterized by broken hairs of varying length. Within the patches, hair loss is not complete. Some children with trichotillosis also have trichophagy—the habit of eating the hair they pluck. These patients can develop abdominal masses consisting of balls of undigested hair (trichobezoar). Treatment requires behavioral modification and help from a psychologist. As long as the hair trauma was not severe or chronic enough to cause scarring, the hair will regrow when the trauma is stopped.

Telogen effluvium occurs in the setting of chronic disease or recent severe illness, high fever, flu, or severe emotional stress. Hairs that were in their growth phase are suddenly converted into their resting phase. Two to 4 months later, when the child is otherwise well, these hairs can begin to shed. The shedding, which is actually a mass exodus of follicles from growth into resting phase, can last for up to 6 weeks. The hair loss is not total nor does it tend to show up in patches. It can be significant and alarming. It typically appears thin throughout the scalp. Unless the initial cause is repeated, all of the hairs normally return (the classic case of telogen effluvium is postpartum hair loss). No blood work is necessary for this type of hair loss. Parents and children can be reassured that the child will not become completely bald and that hair will start to regrow within a few months. It is important to tell parents that often the texture and density of the hair may be different when hair regrows. Patients may never regain the density they had initially. Lead levels can be evaluated in children with diffuse or patchy hair loss if suspicion is high.

Scarring alopecia is rare in children, and the differential diagnosis includes discoid lupus, sarcoidosis, and lichen planopilaris. In each of these diseases, the alopecic skin looks scarred (smooth and shiny with no evidence of hair follicles). A biopsy is necessary to help differentiate these so these patients should be referred to a dermatologist.

Summary

A few simple questions can help differentiate the most common types of nonscarring hair loss, although a few disease can present in different categories. Generally, the pathway in Figure 14-3 will help guide initial diagnostic work-up.

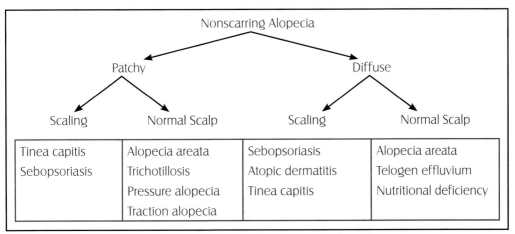

Figure 41-3. Schema for differentiating types of nonscarring alopecia.

Suggested Readings

Alkhalifah A, Alsantali A, Wang E, McElwee KJ, Shapirom J. Alopecia areata update: part II. Treatment. *J Am Acad Dermatol.* 2010;62(2):191-202.

Mohrenschlager M, Seidl HP, Ring J, Abeck D. Pediatric tinea capitis: recognition and management. *Am J Clin Dermatol.* 2005;6(4):203-213.

Mukherjee N, Burkhart CN, Morrell DS. Treatment of alopecia areata in children. *Pediatr Ann.* 2009;38(7):388-395.

Rushton DH. Nutritional factors and hair loss. *Clin Exp Dermatol.* 2002;27(5):396-404.

Slonim AE, Sadick N, Pugliese M, Meyers-Seifer CH. Clinical response of alopecia, trichorrheix nodosa and dry scaly skin to zinc supplementation. *J Pediatr.* 1992;121(6):890-895.

Tay YK, Levy ML, Metry DW. Trichotillomania in childhood: case series and review. *Pediatrics.* 2004;113(5):e494-e498.

Trost LB, Bergfeld WF, Calogeras E. The diagnosis and treatment of iron deficiency and its potential relationship to hair loss. *J Am Acad Dermatol.* 2006;54(5):824-844.

SECTION VII

ACNE

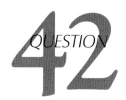

WHAT ARE THE DIFFERENT TYPES OF ACNE AND HOW IS EACH TYPE TREATED?

Magdalene Dohil, MD and Lawrence F. Eichenfield, MD

There are several types of acne seen in children presenting at different ages: infantile acne, midchildhood acne, preadolescent, and adolescent acne. Neonatal acne is a more complicated term, as discussed below.

Neonatal Acne

The term *neonatal acne* is traditionally used to describe a broad set of pustular eruptions in neonates that are self-limited. Most of the time, these eruptions are not really acneiform, and do not have comedones (whiteheads and blackheads) or acneiform inflammatory lesions. The term *neonatal cephalic pustulosis* has been used to define erythematous papules and pustules on the face, neck, scalp, and torso presenting in the first weeks of life. This may be associated with colonization or infection with *Malassezia* species (*M sympodialis* and *M globosa*) in some, but not all, patients although it remains controversial whether the *Malassezia* is pathogenic. The condition is self-limited and many families and physicians choose not to treat with any medication. For those who prefer treatment, prompt response is often noted with antiyeast agents, such as ketoconazole. Some neonates actually present with comedonal acne. These infants may have a more prolonged course, overlapping with the more typical presentation of infantile acne, and can be managed in the same manner discussed below.

Infantile Acne

Infantile acne is more commonly characterized by classic comedonal lesions as well as papules, pustules, and occasionally cysts, nodules, and scars (Figure 42-1). It can begin in the first few months of life and persist for months to years. Most of the time, there is no

Figure 42-1. Nodular acne on the cheek of a 2 year old with areas of xerosis from overwashing.

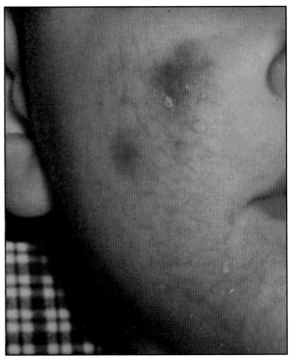

specific endocrinopathy associated with it. However, it would be prudent to assess the infant for signs of abnormal growth, androgenizing signs, precocious puberty, or other atypical clinical features that might suggest the utility of an endocrinologic evaluation.

Standard approaches to treatment include topical medicines including benzoyl peroxide, retinoids, antibiotics, and combination therapies. While these agents form the mainstay of therapy, systemic treatments such as oral antibiotics (of course not with a tetracycline agent!) and even isotretinoin should be considered in rare severe and recalcitrant cases. For the more severe cases that might require systemic therapy, referral to dermatology is reasonable.

Mid-Childhood Acne

Mid-childhood acne, acne in 1 to 7 year olds, is essentially acne vulgaris (common acne) in an age group where it is very uncommon and usually associated with significant pathology. Acne in this age group can be related to premature adrenarche, Cushing syndrome, congenital adrenal hyperplasia, gonadal/adrenal tumors, and true precocious puberty. Children should be evaluated with tanner staging; a growth chart to assess rapid gains in height percentile that may be seen in androgen excess or weight percentiles going up and height down in Cushing Syndrome; bone age; and hormonal evaluation including total/free testosterone, dehydroepiandrosterone sulfate, androstenedione, and perhaps luteinizing hormone, follicle-stimulating hormone, prolactin, and 17-OH progesterone levels. Referral to pediatric endocrinology is recommended as well. Skin findings presumed to be acne may not infrequently be mistaken for a variety of other conditions, including keratosis pilaris, milia, rosacea, periorificial dermatitis, and *Demodex*. Treatment with topical benzoyl peroxide, retinoids, antibiotics, and combinations of these is reasonable, and oral medications may be utilized for more severe cases. However, it should be noted that tetracyclines should not be used in patients less than 8 years of age.

Preadolescent and Adolescent Acne

Acne can be the first signs of puberty, generally correlating with adrenarche, which correlates with increased sebum production on the face, chest, and trunk (the acne prone areas) and colonization with *Propionibacterium acnes*, the anaerobic bacteria that colonizes the sebaceous follicles and is involved in acne pathogenesis. Often in the preadolescent, facial comedones are predominant, especially on the forehead and central face, and truncal acne is uncommon. More significant comedonal acne in early teenage years is predictive of more severe acne in the future, so being attentive to early acne is recommended.

Factors to be considered in evaluating acne include the predominant lesion type comedones (whiteheads/blackheads), inflammatory papules/pustules, nodules or cyst-like lesions, the extent of the acne (mild, moderate, severe), presence or absence of scarring, and any psychological impact the acne may have on the individual.

Initial therapy for mild acne should include topical medications, such as benzoyl peroxide, retinoids (adapalene, tretinoin, tazarotene), antibiotics (clindamycin, erythromycin), or combination therapy. Moderate acne usually requires a topical retinoid, with either topical antimicrobials or an oral antibiotic. Benzoyl peroxide is usually advised in a regimen with topical or oral antibiotics to minimize the development of bacterial resistance. Unresponsive cases may require gradual increases in strength of retinoids, and additions of other topical agents not being utilized, oral antibiotics, hormonal therapy in older adolescent females, and isotretinoin.

Suggested Readings

Ayhan M, Sancak B, Karaduman A, Arikan S, Sahin S. Colonization of neonate skin by *Malassezia* species: relationship with neonatal cephalic pustulosis. *J Am Acad Dermatol.* 2007;57(6):1012-1018. Epub 2007 Sep 24.

Bergman JN, Eichenfield LF. Neonatal acne and cephalic pustulosis: is malassezia the whole story? *Arch Dermatol.* 2002;138(2:255-257.

Kroshinsky D, Glick SA. Pediatric rosacea. *Dermatol Ther.* 2006;19(4):196-201.

Lucky AW, Biro FM, Huster GA, Leach AD, Morrison JA, Ratterman J. Acne vulgaris in premenarchal girls. An early sign of puberty associated with rising levels of dehydroepiandrosterone. *Arch Dermatol.* 1994;130(3):308-314.

Lucky AW, Biro FM, Huster GA, Morrison JA, Elder N. Acne vulgaris in early adolescent boys. Correlations with pubertal maturation and age. *Arch Dermatol.* 1991;127(2):210-216.

Mourelatos K, Eady EA, Cunliffe WJ, Clark SM, Cove JH. Temporal changes in sebum excretion and propionibacterial colonization in preadolescent children with and without acne. *Br J Dermatol.* 2007;156(1):22-31.

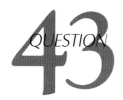

WHAT IS A REASONABLE AMOUNT OF TIME TO TREAT ACNE BEFORE THE PATIENT IS REFERRED TO A DERMATOLOGIST?

Marissa J. Perman, MD

Acne vulgaris is a chronic and sometimes frustrating inflammatory condition of the pilosebaceous unit that usually begins during puberty. The pathophysiology of acne is multifactorial and related to follicular epithelial hyperproliferation and keratinization, inflammation, excess sebum production, and *Propionibacterium acnes* (*P acnes*) infection of the follicle. Understanding the pathogenesis, classification, and severity of the acne will help guide your therapeutic options. In addition, knowing each therapy's time to maximal efficacy will help direct you on when to try alternative therapies versus when to refer.

In general, acne is characterized as primary lesions, which can be noninflammatory; composed of open and closed comedones (blackheads and whiteheads, respectively); and inflammatory lesions, which include papules, pustules, and nodules. Many of these lesions will resolve without a permanent scar, but patients whose primary lesions leave scars may benefit from early dermatologic consultation.

For primarily mild comedonal acne, topical retinoids are the mainstay of treatment. For mild inflammatory or mixed acne (a combination of comedones and inflammatory papules or pustules), products with benzoyl peroxide or a combination topical benzoyl peroxide-antibiotic (such as benzoyl peroxide-clindamycin) preparation in addition to retinoids offer a good starting point. Retinoids normalize follicular hyperproliferation, which causes follicular plugging, as well as decrease inflammation. Benzoyl peroxide is antimicrobial and keratolytic. Antibiotics are anti-inflammatory and antimicrobial. I recommend starting with lower strength retinoids for most patients as they tend to be irritating for the first 1 to 3 weeks. I council my patients to expect 50% to 75% improvement after 12 weeks.

If there is no significant improvement after 3 to 4 months, I increase the strength of the retinoid or try a different topical antibiotic or other combination product. If there is still

Figure 43-1. Comedonal acne on the cheek with some inflammatory papules.

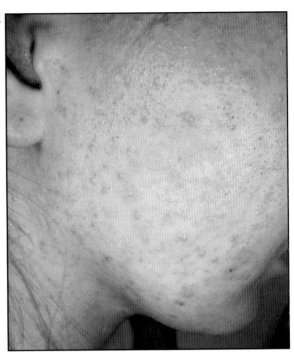

no improvement by 6 months, I move on to therapy for moderate acne (see next). Other topical therapies that can be considered in the early stages of treatment include salicylic acid, azelaic acid, and sulfur-containing products.

For moderate acne (Figure 43-1), there are several treatment pathways available. Topical therapy for moderate comedonal, inflammatory, or mixed acne as described previously is still a reasonable place to start, as many compliant patients will have success with topical therapy alone. My first choice for patients with more severe moderate acne includes a combination of topical therapy in combination with oral antibiotics. I generally start with a topical retinoid and an oral tetracycline, usually doxycycline if the child is over 8 years old. In addition, I may also prescribe a topical benzoyl peroxide-antibiotic preparation. Remember that one of the risks of tetracyclines is staining of growing teeth and bones. Children over 8 years may have all of their secondary teeth (except molars, which are less visible and thus staining is less of a problem) but there are many children who develop more slowly. Therefore, tetracyclines may still cause tooth staining in any child who does not have all of his or her secondary teeth especially since therapy for acne can often last months. Minocycline is often used for acne, but I typically choose doxycycline as first line because minocycline has more of a risk of causing a lupus-like reaction, severe drug hypersensitivity including Stevens-Johnson syndrome, pseudotumor cerebri, and blue skin pigmentation especially in acne scars.[1] Oral antibiotics for acne, similar to topical antibiotics, are important for both their anti-inflammatory effects and inhibition of *P acnes*. Improvement should not be expected for at least 8 to 12 weeks, and significant resolution can take up to 4 to 6 months. Oral antibiotics for acne are often necessary to prevent severe scarring and social distress. But, long-term antibiotic use may lead to resistance, and there are emerging reports suggesting a link between tetracycline use in acne with inflammatory bowel disease.[2]

Hormonal therapy is another important treatment option for moderate acne. Patients who report flares of their acne just before or during menses likely have a hormonal component. In addition, patients with polycystic ovarian syndrome (PCOS) often develop hormonal-related acne. For these patients, it is reasonable to consider monotherapy with an oral contraceptive pill (OCP). The three OCPs FDA approved for acne vulgaris are drospirenone (Yaz), norethindrone (Estrostep), and norgestimate (Ortho-Tricylen); however, many combination OCPs provide benefits despite lack of FDA approval.

In some patients with mild-to-moderate acne with a hormonal component, it is appropriate to start with the more traditional therapy described above, particularly topical therapy, and then add OCPs if needed. I often base this decision on patient and parent preferences. Some patients are better at taking a daily pill than applying topical therapies and will opt for this therapy. Other patients and families are reluctant to start OCPs because their primary indication is for birth control. OCPs should be continued for several months before assessing response.

Additional hormonal therapies include antiandrogen medications such as spironolactone, a combination antiandrogen and aldosterone medication. Spironolactone is not FDA approved to treat acne vulgaris; however, dermatologists have used this medication successfully to treat hormone-related acne as well as hirsutism, often seen together in PCOS. Spironolactone has several possible side effects, most notably hypotension, hyperkalemia, breast tenderness, and menstrual irregularities and should only be used by providers comfortable managing these and other side effects. Patients should be counseled about birth control as spironolactone is pregnancy category C. In addition, patients should be informed of the black box warning regarding a tumorigenic potential found in rats receiving high doses of a compound similar to spironolactone.

Referral to dermatology should be considered for patients with unresponsive or minimally responsive mild-to-moderate acne despite adjustments to the potency of the topical retinoid, alternating topical antibiotics with or without benzoyl peroxide, and switching the oral antibiotic within the tetracycline class. The time frame varies but generally should be anywhere from 6 to 12 months after initiating therapy.

There are several reasons not to delay referral. First, patients with moderate and occasionally mild acne, comedonal or inflammatory, can develop scarring at any time (Figure 43-2). Scarring acne is often an indication for more aggressive therapy such as isotretinoin and should be started sooner rather than later to avoid further irreversible damage. Another concern is the risk of antibiotic resistance with long-term antibiotic use. Patients with moderate acne who fail conventional antibiotics used in acne after several months should also see a dermatologist for alternative options such as isotretinoin.

Patients with severe nodular acne or moderate inflammatory acne with scarring at the first visit should be referred to a dermatologist immediately for possible isotretinoin therapy. In the meantime, therapy for moderate inflammatory acne should be initiated until the patient is seen by a dermatologist. This includes an OCP if there is a hormonal component as most adolescent females on isotretinoin will also be placed on an OCP. Some patients who appear to be isotretinoin candidates prior to starting an OCP may not require isotretinoin after the OCP is started.

Acne management reflects the art of medicine and must be individualized for each patient. Figure 43-3 summarizes my general guidelines on acne management. When in doubt, it is better to refer sooner rather than later as acne can have a significant psychosocial impact on patients when not managed appropriately.

Figure 43-2. Moderate to severe acne on the back with scarring.

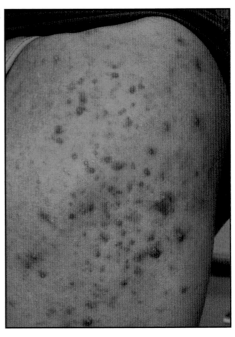

Figure 43-3. Basic algorithm for acne management. (BP indicates benzoyl peroxide; OCP, oral contraceptive pills)

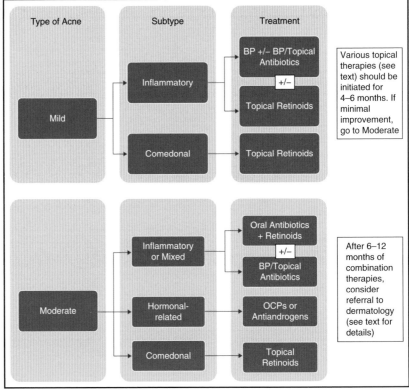

References

1. Strauss JS, Krowchuk DP, Leyden JJ, Lucky AW, Shalita AR, Siegfried EC, Thiboutot DM, Van Voorhees AS, Beutner KA, Sieck CK, Bhushan R; American Academy of Dermatology/American Academy of Dermatology Association. Guidelines of care for acne vulgaris management. *J Am Acad Dermatol.* 2007;56(4):651-663.
2. Margolis DJ, Fanelli M, Hoffstad O, Lewis JD. Potential association between the oral tetracycline class of antimicrobials used to treat acne and inflammatory bowel disease. *Am J Gastroenterol.* 2010;105(12):2610-2616. Epub 2010 Aug 10.

Suggested Readings

Eichenfield LF, Fowler JF Jr, Fried RG, Friedlander SF, Levy ML, Webster GF. Perspectives on therapeutic options for acne: an update. *Semin Cutan Med Surg.* 2010;29(2 Suppl 1):13-16.
Junkins-Hopkins JM. Hormone therapy for acne. *J Am Acad Dermatol.* 2010;62(3):486-488.

SECTION VIII

OTHER

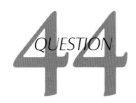

44

HOW CAN I MANAGE HIDRADENITIS SUPPURATIVA?

Adam Nabatian, MD and Warren R. Heymann, MD

Hidradenitis suppurativa (HS) is a common chronic recurrent multifocal disease of skin and subcutaneous tissues affecting flexural areas where it causes inflammation, scarring, and sinus formation (Figure 44-1). HS is a debilitating follicular skin disease where pain and the discharge of pus from sinus tracts causes significant morbidity.[1] Diagnosis relies on recognition of the inflammatory lesions in the apocrine gland-bearing areas of the body, most commonly in the axillary, inguinal, and anogenital regions. HS typically begins after puberty. The primary mechanism in the disease is thought to be occlusion of the follicle in the pilosebaceous infundibulum followed by its rupture with subsequent inflammation.[2] The disease is often associated with other members of the so-called "follicular occlusion tetrad"—acne conglobata, dissecting cellulitis of the scalp, and a pilonidal cyst.

HS adversely affects a patient's quality of life; recent studies have confirmed that this is especially true for patients with anogenital lesions. Patients with lesions on exposed skin may feel stigmatized. Many physicians and other health care providers may be perplexed and frustrated when a patient presents with HS since it is difficult to treat and patients are often left with unsatisfactory clinical results.

The first step in treating patients with HS is to be confident of the diagnosis. Other diagnostic considerations include bacterial furunculosis, secondarily infected epidermoid cysts, inflammatory bowel disease (especially Crohn's disease), and rarely other entities such as cutaneous tuberculosis, atypical mycobacterial infections, or amebiasis. Cultures and occasionally skin biopsies may be of value, especially if one is concerned about the possibility of the development of a squamous cell carcinoma, which may be a rare complication of HS. A very rare complication of HS, but one to be remembered, is secondary amyloidosis, due to tissue accumulation of the reactant serum amyloid A; this can deposit in many organs, resulting in problems such as nephrotic syndrome.

Lesions in HS are divided into three stages.[1] In stage one lesions, typically deep and rounded boils are present. Stage two lesions demonstrate scarring and sinus formation in separate areas of the affected regions. In stage three lesions, scarring and sinuses coalesce.[1] Early lesions, prior to the appearance of scars and sinus tracts, are more responsive to

Figure 44-1. Axilla showing scarred nodules and sinus tract formation indicative of chronic disease.

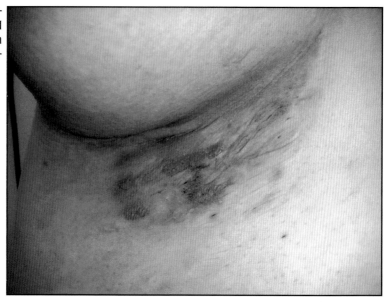

therapy. Once sinus tracts appear, the treatment options are more limited. Therefore, therapy must target patients as early as possible in the course of their illness, with the goal of preventing scarring and sinus tract formation, if possible.

Treating HS is complicated, and one should approach the disease from the perspective of the "therapeutic ladder," beginning with the safest medications that may offer some benefit (Table 44-1). A multimodality approach is often necessary to get patients in remission. One should not forget about attempting to ameliorate aggravating factors. Encourage the patient to wear comfortable clothing. Weight loss is advised in obese patients since this may help with the treatment of HS by reducing the pressure and shearing forces at the affected sites.

Initial treatment utilizes topical medications. We prefer to use topical clindamycin on early lesions because patients frequently respond to treatment and there has been research studies demonstrating its efficacy.[1] Azelaic acid cream may be added to the antibiotic regimen as a regional prophylactic treatment. Decolonization strategies similar to those used in patients with methicillin-resistant *Staphylococcus aureus* infections may be of value.

Systemic treatments are often necessary. Some physicians use systemic tetracycline 500 mg orally twice daily as an alternative to topical antibiotics; however, systemic therapy with tetracycline did not show better results than with topical therapy with clindamycin.[3] Despite that, there may be an anti-inflammatory value to the use of one of the tetracyclines (tetracycline, doxycycline, or minocycline) for patients with inflammatory lesions of HS. Superinfections of HS lesions may be treated with oral clindamycin 300 mg twice daily or dicloxacillin 500 mg three times daily but therapy should be directed by bacterial cultures. Hormonal therapy with cyproterone acetate may be helpful for some females; however, there are many safety concerns with this treatment since it requires high doses, continued use, and may not be available in all areas. For inflammatory disease, dapsone may be of value. Although oral retinoids, such as isotretinoin, seem appealing on a theoretical basis, they have had little benefit in HS. Biologic agents

Table 44-1
Treatment Options for Mild, Moderate, and Severe Hidradenitis Suppurativa

Severity of Hidradenitis Suppurativa	Treatment Options
Mild	• Topical clindamycin and/or azelaic acid • Oral tetracyclines (tetracycline, doxycycline, or minocycline)
Moderate	• Intralesional corticosteroids • Localized excision of sinus tracts • "Deroofing" technique
Severe	• Excision of the affected tissue • Laying open of all the sinus tracts • Dapsone • Oral retinoids • TNF-alpha inhibitors

TNF indicates tumor necrosis factor

(notably the tumor necrosis factor-alpha inhibitors etanercept, adalimumab, infliximab) have shown promise but require further testing to demonstrate safety and efficacy.[4] Although immunosuppressive agents such as cyclosporine have been reported to be effective in some case reports, we would only consider this option as a last resort, for short-term use.

Intralesional corticosteroids or localized excisions of sinus tracts are often very valuable. The "deroofing" technique, a tissue-saving procedure where the "roof" of an abscess, cyst, or sinus tract is electrosurgically removed, is an effective minimally invasive intervention for the treatment of mild-to-moderate HS lesions at fixed locations.[2] With the surgical deroofing technique, there is a limited recurrence and good long-term results.[2]

The most definitive treatment involves major surgery. Surgical intervention involves excision of the affected tissue or laying open of all sinus tracts.[1] Surgical procedures may be very extensive, and healing may either be by primary or secondary intention, depending on the extent of disease. Patients need to be prepared for a prolonged convalescence following extensive surgery. Perhaps the newer "deroofing" technique will enable some patients to regain a reasonable quality of life more quickly than traditional surgery.

Despite the many challenges confronting patients with HS, a compassionate physician attuned to the psychosocial stresses that afflict patients with the disease, combined with a rational, multifaceted therapeutic plan, can bring a reasonable level of comfort to these individuals.

References

1. Jemec GBE. Hidradenitis suppurativa. In: Lebwohl MG, Heymann WR, Berth-Jones J, Coulson I, eds. *Treatment of Skin Disease: Comprehensive Therapeutic Strategies.* 2nd ed. Philadelphia, PA: Mosby; 2006:280-281.
2. van der Zee HH, Prens EP, Boer J. Deroofing: a tissue-saving technique for the treatment of mild to moderate hidradenitis suppurativa lesions. *J Am Acad Dermatol.* 2010;63(3):475-480.
3. Jemec GB, Wendelboe P. Topical clindamycin versus systemic tetracycline in the treatment of hidradenitis suppurativa. *J Am Acad Dermatol.* 1998;39(6):971-974.
4. Adams DR, Yankura JA, Fogelberg AC, Anderson BE. Treatment of hidradenitis suppurativa with etanercept injection. *Arch Dermatol.* 2010;146(5):501-504.

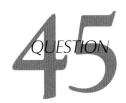

WHEN SHOULD I SUSPECT AND HOW DO I MANAGE HAIR PULLING (TRICHOTILLOMANIA)?

Marissa J. Perman, MD

Trichotillomania (TTM) is a relatively common cause of alopecia from the conscious or unconscious habit of pulling one's hair. Unless hair pulling is suspected, it can easily be mistaken for other causes of alopecia. TTM affects an estimated 1% of the population, although this may be an underestimate due to missed diagnoses from secretive patient behaviors and the difficulty in consistently defining TTM. Hair pulling usually begins either in early childhood or adolescence.[1] In children, TTM occurs equally in both genders, and older children may exhibit other compulsive behaviors such as nail biting or skin picking.

The *Diagnostic and Statistical Manual of Mental Disorders, Fourth Edition Text Revision* (DSM-IV-TR; American Psychiatric Association, 2000) classifies TTM as an impulse control disorder not otherwise specified. The strict criteria for TTM for both adults and children can be found in the DSM-IV-TR. Some believe the criteria are too strict as many patients deny feeling a sense of tension before or gratification after pulling their hair, and "noticeable hair loss" may be open to interpretation. Instead, TTM may be better classified as an anxiety disorder because it is associated with features of obsessive-compulsive disorder.[2]

Hair pulling in younger children (age <8 years) is often a benign, self-limited behavior that resolves over time without intervention. A sense of tension or anxiety before or gratification following hair pulling is unlikely in this age group. In older children and adults, two forms of hair pulling include automatic and focused hair pulling. The automatic type consists of unconscious hair pulling while the child is involved in another task such as watching television, doing homework, lying in bed, or talking on the telephone. The focused type is associated with awareness of the act in response to an impulse or increasing tension, is seen more commonly in adolescents, and appears to be associated with stress or anxiety. A combination of automatic and focused hair pulling is seen in many older children and adults.[1]

Clinically, several clues will aid you in the diagnosis. The scalp is the most common site of involvement. Eyelashes and eyebrows are the next most commonly involved sites, but any hair-bearing site such as genital or nasal hair can be affected. One or multiple sites may be involved at any one time. In a retrospective review of 10 children with TTM, the most common scalp sites involved included frontal and vertex, followed by parietal, occipital, and temporal scalp.[2] Classic findings include well-defined, linear, or angular patches of alopecia that are never completely bald and contain scattered, broken hairs of varying lengths. Perifollicular erythema or excoriations may also be present.

Trichophagia (ingestion of hair) is found in 5% to 18% of patients with TTM and can lead to trichobezoar (hairball) and its associated complications.[2] In addition, many children partake in bizarre oral behaviors such as touching or tickling their lips or nose with the hair once pulled.

The differential diagnosis includes alopecia areata, tinea capitis, and syphilis. Alopecia areata can be distinguished by its smooth, round patches of complete alopecia in one or multiple locations on the scalp. Eyebrows and eyelashes may also be involved. Exclamation point hairs (hairs with a tapered end) may be found at the periphery of an alopecic patch. Alopecia areata occasionally proceeds TTM.[2] Tinea capitis is often associated with erythema and scale, and hairs in the affected region break easily as opposed to the hair in TTM. A potassium hydroxide mount or fungal culture should be obtained if the diagnosis is uncertain. The alopecia associated with syphilis is described as "moth-eaten" with patchy diffuse alopecia. These patients may also have other findings of secondary syphilis such as the papulosquamous eruption on the trunk and brown macules on the palms and soles. Serologic testing for syphilis is diagnostic. If a clinical diagnosis of TTM cannot be made, a scalp biopsy may be helpful. Histologic evidence of TTM includes increased catagen and telogen hairs, pigmented hair casts, follicular plugging, and empty hair ducts.

Management of TTM is challenging and requires sensitivity and patience. A strong patient-physician relationship with parental support is ideal. I suggest avoiding direct confrontation as many patients will deny hair pulling when accused. Gently introducing the possibility that the patient may be pulling his or her hair and may or may not be aware of the action is the best approach. This should be followed by obtaining more information about associated home and/or school stressors that may have led to the behavior.

Younger children (<8 years) often do not need therapy as the behavior is self-limited. As for prepubertal and adolescent patients, reassurance and support are the most important factors for eliminating TTM. This can be supplemented with behavioral therapy or counseling for both the patient and the family, which is successful in many cases. For patients with significant psychopathology such as anxiety, depression, or obsessive-compulsive disorder, psychiatry referral is important. Selective serotonin reuptake inhibitors, tricyclic antidepressants, and antipsychotics have all been tried with varying success and may be more successful in conjunction with behavioral therapy. The dose may need to be adjusted based on weight in children.

N-acetylcysteine, an amino acid thought to restore extracellular glutamate concentrations in the nucleus accumbens (the part of the brain that deals with reward and addiction), may play a role in treating repetitive and compulsive behaviors. A double-blind, placebo-controlled study evaluating N-acetylcysteine in 50 adult patients with TTM was recently published. The patients in the N-acetylcysteine group received 1200 mg/day for 6 weeks followed by 2400 mg/day for 6 weeks. The authors concluded that 56% of the patients receiving N-acetylcysteine reported "much" or "very much" improvement in their disease symptoms versus 16% in the placebo group following 12 weeks of treatment

(P = 0.003).[3] Further studies are needed, but this may offer another safe pharmacotherapeutic approach in conjunction with behavioral therapy.

Including the patient, family, and teachers in the care plan is important for successful management of TTM, particularly in older children. Children are often motivated to discontinue their hair-pulling behaviors but need support and guidance from the adults in their life. The Trichotillomania Learning Center, accessible by Web site at www.trich.org, contains a wealth of information and support for patients, parents, and providers.[4]

References

1. Duke DC, Keeley ML, Geffken GR, Storch EA. Trichotillomania: a current review. *Clin Psychol Rev.* 2010;30(2): 181-193. Epub 2009 Oct 30.
2. Tay YK, Levy ML, Metry DW. Trichotillomania in childhood: case series and review. *Pediatrics.* 2004;113(5): e494-e498.
3. Grant JE, Odlaug BL, Kim SW. N-acetylcysteine, a glutamate modulator, in the treatment of trichotillomania: a double-blind, placebo-controlled study. *Arch Gen Psychiatry.* 2009;66(7):756-763.
4. Mansueto CS, Ninan PT, Rothbaum BO, Reeve E. Trichotillomania and its treatment in children and adolescents: a guide for clinicians. http://www.trich.org/dnld/Child_Clinicians_Guide_v08.pdf. Accessed January 28, 2011.

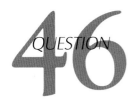

HOW SHOULD I MANAGE HYPERHIDROSIS?

Randy Tang, MD and Warren R. Heymann, MD

Hyperhidrosis, defined as sweating in excess of what is required for thermoregulation, affects approximately 3% of the population. It can either be generalized or localized to a certain part of the body, especially areas with a high concentration of sweat glands like the palms, soles, axillae, and groin. This debilitating condition interferes with all aspects of an affected individual's life often causing social embarrassment in addition to physical complications such as the potential for dehydration and skin infections. Patients with hyperhidrosis of the palms complain of difficulty performing routine activities that require a dry hand or firm grasp, such as performing schoolwork or playing sports. Individuals with hyperhidrosis of the axillae often will limit their arm movements just to hide sweat spots and in many cases will change their clothing several times a day. Finally, patients often report that they get nervous when they sweat, and subsequently sweat more because they are nervous, further exacerbating their symptoms.

Hyperhidrosis can be classified as either a primary disorder or secondary to another medical condition. Primary hyperhidrosis, which may be inherited as an autosomal dominant trait, appears around the onset of puberty and is believed to be due to sympathetic overactivity. Secondary hyperhidrosis occurs in the setting of another medical condition, usually due to a neurological, infectious, or endocrine disorder (Table 46-1). This review will focus on the management of primary hyperhidrosis because the treatment for secondary hyperhidrosis is targeted at managing the underlying condition or removing the underlying cause.

A good history and physical examination, along with some laboratory work including a basic metabolic panel and thyroid function studies, is the first step in evaluating a patient with hyperhidrosis and will often help distinguish whether a patient has a primary or secondary process. For example, night sweats can be associated with an underlying malignancy. Therefore, it would be prudent to obtain a full blood count as part of the work-up. A patient with episodic flushing should raise the suspicion for hyperthyroidism or carcinoid syndrome, and obtaining a 24-hour urinary excretion of 5-hydroxyindolacetic acid (5-HIAA) and thyroid-stimulating hormone level could be appropriate. On the other hand, a patient with sustained or paroxysmal hypertension in conjunction with

---

Table 46-1

Causes of Secondary Hyperhidrosis

General Causes

Anxiety
Exercise
Febrile Illness

Cardiac/Hematological Causes

Congestive heart failure
Porphyria

Endocrine Causes

Acromegaly
Diabetes mellitus
Hyperthyroidism
Menopausal state
Pregnancy

Infectious Causes

HIV
Tuberculosis
Endocarditis

Malignancy-Related Causes

Carcinoid syndrome
Glomus tumor
Myeloproliferative disorders
Pheochromocytoma

Neurological Causes

Peripheral neuropathy
Parkinson disease
Spinal cord injury
Syringomyelia

Substance Induced

Alcohol withdrawal
Cholinesterase Inhibitors
Opioids
SSRIs
Tricyclic antidepressants

Miscellaneous Causes

Blue rubber bleb nevus
Burning feet syndrome
Complex regional pain syndrome
Gout
Harlequin syndrome
Familial dysautonomia
Parotid gland surgery (Frey syndrome)
POEMS syndrome
Shapiro syndrome
Speckled lentiginous nevus syndrome

---

hyperhidrosis should be worked up for pheochromocytomas or paragangliomas by testing for plasma and urinary metanephrines. Although tests are not required to confirm the presence of primary hyperhidrosis, the application of starch and iodine to skin areas with hyperhidrosis can help define the areas of maximum sweating.

The management of primary hyperhidrosis involves both lifestyle modifications and medical intervention (Figure 46-1). Patients should be counseled to avoid factors or triggers that exacerbate their hyperhidrosis, including anxiety-provoking situations, caffeinated foods and drinks, and nicotine. Therapeutic options for managing primary hyperhidrosis include topical therapies, oral medications, iontophoresis, botulinum toxin A, and surgery (Table 46-2).

Topical over-the-counter antiperspirants containing aluminum chlorohydrate (AC) or prescription strength antiperspirants containing aluminum chloride hexahydrate (ACH) 20% to 25% in alcohol are recommended as first-line treatments for hyperhidrosis.[1] Aluminum chloride compounds appear to work by occluding the intraepidermal eccrine duct below the level of the stratum corneum. The solution should be applied to the unshaven axillae nightly and washed off in the morning. In some patients who fail to respond to standard ACH in an alcohol base, a different preparation using 4% salicylic

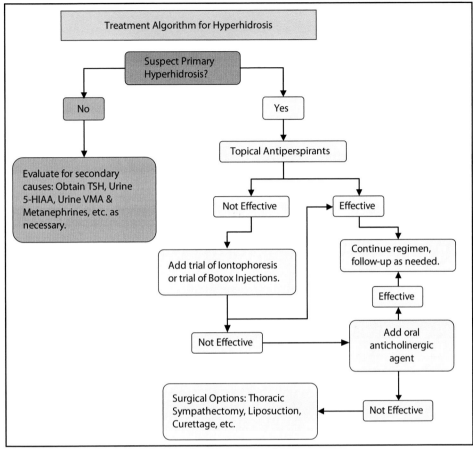

Figure 46-1. Treatment algorithm for hyperhidrosis.

Table 46-2	
Treatment Options for Primary Hyperhidrosis	
Topical agents	Aluminum chlorohydrate, aluminum chloride hexahydrate (+/− 4% salicylic acid), topical glycopyrrolate
Oral agents	Glycopyrrolate, propantheline bromide, oxybutynin, rarely: clonidine, diltiazem
Injections	Botulinum toxin A
Surgical options	Thoracic sympathectomy ("open" or "minimally invasive/endoscopic" approach), liposuction, curettage
Other	Iontophoresis

acid in a hydroalcoholic gel base as a vehicle for the ACH has been shown to be effective.[2] An oral anticholinergic agent such as 1 mg of sodium glycopyrrolate taken 45 minutes before application of ACH may also help increase the efficacy of ACH by reducing sweating at the time of application but this can produce severe side effects and is rarely used in children. This allows the ACH to be retained on the skin and exert its effect on the sweat pores.[1] It may take up to 3 weeks before a patient notices improvement. Some individuals experience skin irritation because AC/ACH in the presence of moisture forms hydrochloric acid. In these individuals, a mild topical corticosteroid can reduce this unwanted side effect. Rarely, AC or ACH cause an allergic contact dermatitis, in which case another treatment modality should be considered.

Iontophoresis, a process that introduces salt ions in solution through the skin, is another treatment option available for pediatric hyperhidrosis sufferers, especially those with palmoplantar hyperhidrosis. A patient's hands or feet are placed into 2 trays filled with tap water in one of several commercially available devices for 20 minutes 3 times a week. A current is passed through the trays via two electrodes present in the water until the patient experiences some slight discomfort. Although the mechanism of how iontophoresis reduces sweating is currently unknown, patients often report improvement in their symptoms after a few treatments. Patients typically experience a recurrence of symptoms with treatment cessation. Iontophoresis is contraindicated in patients who are pregnant and in those individuals who have cardiac pacemakers or metal implants.

For more severe hyperhidrosis sufferers, botulinum toxin A (produced by the anerobic bacterium *Clostridium botulinum*), injected intradermally into the axillae or palms, produces sustained anhidrosis for several months by irreversibly blocking the release of acetylcholine from cholinergic junctions.[3] While inactivation of affected cholinergic junctions is permanent, the effect is temporary because new cholinergic junctions are produced through turnover and repair. Injection of botulinum toxin into palmar skin is less well tolerated compared to the axillae and, therefore, may require a regional wrist anesthetic blockade. There is also potential for producing weakness of the intrinsic hand muscles with palmar injections.

Anticholinergic agents can be used in more severe hyperhidrosis when the benefits outweigh the risks. Although only studied in adults, these drugs have had success in treating pediatric cases of hyperhidrosis.[2] Oral anticholinergic agents such as sodium glycopyrrolate or propantheline bromide produce a dose-related inhibition of sweating by acting as competitive antagonists of acetylcholine at the muscarinic receptor. Unfortunately, the dose necessary to inhibit sweat production often produces unwanted anticholingergic side effects (dry mouth, pupillary dilatation, photophobia, glaucoma, urinary retention, constipation, and tachycardia). A low-dose formulation in combination with topical antiperspirants is often better tolerated and may be highly efficacious.

Finally, in refractory cases of hyperhidrosis, satisfactory long-term results can be achieved via selective ablation of the sympathetic innervations of the palms, axillae, and soles using electrocautery or laser in an endoscopic or open surgical technique.[4] Sympathectomy is associated with a number of possible side effects, including wound infection, scarring, compensatory hyperhidrosis in other areas of the body, Horner syndrome, pneumothorax, and even intraoperative cardiac arrest. Therefore, this treatment is reserved for treating severe palmar hyperhidrosis after careful consideration for the risks and side effects. The surgery is performed as an upper thoracic sympathectomy of the

T2–T3 ganglia, which is associated with the fewest complications. Pediatric and adolescent patients tend to tolerate the procedure better than adults but this procedure is very rarely warranted. Another surgical technique used to manage axillary hyperhidrosis is liposuction that removes subcutaneous tissue containing sweat glands.

Hyperhidrosis is a detriment to many individual's psychological, social, professional, and physical well-being. Fortunately, early detection and management of hyperhidrosis can dramatically improve the quality of life for these individuals.

References

1. Langtry J. Hyperhidrosis. In: Lebwohl MG, Heymann WR, Berth-Jones J, Coulson I, eds. *Treatment of Skin Disease: Comprehensive Therapeutic Strategies.* 3rd ed. Philadelphia, PA: Mosby; 2010:317-320.
2. Gelbard C, Epstein H, Hebert A. Primary pediatric hyperhidrosis: a review of current treatment options. *Pediatr Derm.* 2008;25(6):591-598.
3. Eisenach JH, Atkinson JL, Fealey RD. Hyperhidrosis: evolving therapies for a well-established phenomenon. *Mayo Clin Proc.* 2005;80(5):657-666.
4. Cohen Z, Shinar D, Levi I, et al. Thoracoscopic upper thoracic sympathectomy for primary palmar hyperhidrosis in children and adolescents. *J Pediatr Surg.* 1995;30(3):471-473.

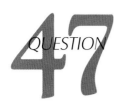

QUESTION

WHAT CAUSES ITCHING WITHOUT ANY RASH?

Dirk M. Elston, MD

Itching unassociated with a rash, or "idiopathic pruritus," has a wide variety of causes, and a systematic approach to the evaluation is helpful. The pathogenesis of itch is complex and involves a sophisticated network of cutaneous nerves, as well as itch-specific mediators and receptors such as interleukin-31 and gastrin-releasing peptide receptor. This question will not be a primer on the basic science of itch. Rather, it will present my approach to the evaluation and treatment of itch unassociated with a primary rash. Common causes include atopic dermatitis, low-grade dermatographism, mastocytosis, xerosis, fiberglass-contaminated clothing, scabies, pediculosis, and tick and mite infestations. Systemic diseases associated with pruritus include renal insufficiency, cholestasis, endocrine and hematologic disorders, internal malignancy, immunobullous diseases, and a variety of acute and chronic infections. Many of these are less common in children than in adults.

The history of onset, duration, intensity, and location of the itch may be helpful clues to the correct diagnosis. Provoking factors such as scratching, heat, pressure, and wool clothing may also be helpful, as may a family history of itch or skin disease. Usually, the diagnosis in a child can be established by history and physical examination, but the evaluation may sometimes require laboratory studies or a skin biopsy for histology or direct immunofluorescence.

When examining the patient, changes caused by scratching should not be misinterpreted as a primary skin rash. Lichenification (an accentuation of the normal skin markings; Figure 47-1), excoriations (scratch marks), prurigo nodularis (picker's nodules; Figure 47-2), crusting as a result of secondary infection, and pigmentary change may all be the result of scratching and should not be interpreted as a primary skin rash. One important clue is that changes that result from scratching only occur at sites that the patient can reach and thus the central back is typically spared.

Primary Cutaneous Disease Associated With Itch

The fundamental problem in atopic dermatitis is a pathologic itch that drives the patient to scratch. Rather than representing a rash that itches, atopic dermatitis has been described as the "itch that rashes." Common skin changes include cheek and extensor

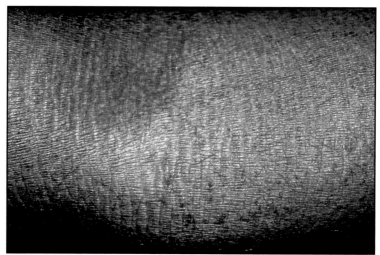

Figure 47-1. Lichenification.

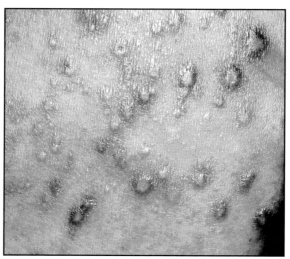

Figure 47-2. Prurigo nodularis.

involvement in young children and flexural lichenification in older children, excoriation, the presence of Dennie-Morgan folds (a double crease under the eyes), pityriasis alba (slightly hypopigmented patches), white dermatographism (a blanch in response to scratching), intolerance to wool clothing, xerosis, and keratosis pilaris. There is typically a family history of atopy. Xerosis is most commonly related to an underlying atopic diathesis but may also be related to central heating or mild underlying ichthyosis.

Dermatographism manifests with a hive in an area that has been scratched. The lesions of subtle dermatographism may not be readily apparent. When broad areas have been scratched, the lesions may not be linear.

Mastocytosis typically presents with subtle, faun-colored macules that hive when scratched but systemic mastocytosis may cause itching in the absence of a rash, and a tryptase level can help in diagnosis.

Children who play near construction sites may encounter fiberglass insulation. More commonly, a parent has done insulation work, then washed the contaminated clothing with the family's laundry. The resulting itch may prove intractable until all contaminated articles of clothing have been discarded.

INFESTATIONS AND BITES

Scabies may present with relatively subtle skin lesions, but there is commonly a history of itching involving other family members. The best places to search for burrows include the wrists, ankles, axillae, web spaces, umbilicus, and the face and scalp in infants. The diagnosis should be confirmed by microscopic examination of skin scrapings.

Pediculosis may present with generalized pruritus with no rash or with a subtle morbilliform rash. Larval ticks, especially *Amblyomma* ticks, appear as small specs that may not be noticed at all or may be misinterpreted as small crusts. The most common scenario is a child who has played in leaves or hung clothing on a bush while swimming. Mite infestations commonly relate to pet infestations or the presence of birds or rodents in or near the house. There may be little to no visible rash. Pets should be inspected for signs of dandruff, dermatitis, or hair loss. The house should be inspected for evidence of nesting material in vents and eaves.

Systemic Disease Associated With Itch

Stigmata of renal or hepatic disease may be apparent on examination. Renal pruritus typically presents with unrelenting itch, although symptoms are commonly worse at night. In cholestatic pruritus, symptoms are intermittent and progressive. The itch is typically worse on the hands and feet and under tight-fitting clothing. Hyper or hypothyroidism can lead to a nonspecific generalized itch.

Work-Up

Laboratory testing is usually not required in children with generalized itch, but those with refractory itch and no apparent diagnosis may benefit from a complete blood count with differential, liver and renal function tests, a thyroid-stimulating hormone, blood glucose, and a serum tryptase. Those with peripheral eosinophilia require stool examinations for ova and parasites or serologic evaluation for *Toxocara* species. Skin scrapings are needed to establish a diagnosis of scabies and a skin biopsy for light microscopy or immunofluorescence may be needed to establish a diagnosis of immunobullous disease.

Ideally, management should be directed at a specific diagnosis. General measures include the use of a bland moisturizer. A mild topical corticosteroid such as desonide 0.05% ointment can be used on lichenified or excoriated areas. Avoidance of skin irritants such as wool clothing is advisable. Baths should be cool, and a mild soap or cleanser such as Dove can be used on soiled areas only. A generous coat of a moisturizer should be applied immediately after bathing. White petrolatum is fragrance free and may be useful for those with sensitivity to fragrances. Lotions with 0.25% camphor and menthol, pramoxine, or both can be helpful. Oral antihistamines such as hydroxyzine or diphenhydramine are useful for histamine-mediated itch and for sedation at bedtime. Importantly, antihistamines can have an opposite activating effect in some children, making them more irritable and energetic.

Narrow band ultraviolet B phototherapy can be helpful if the child is old enough to use the appropriate eye protection.

Suggested Readings

Feramisco JD, Berger TG, Steinhoff M. Innovative management of pruritus. *Dermatol Clin.* 2010;28(3):467-478.
Goetz DW. Vitamin D treatment of idiopathic itch, rash, and urticaria/angioedema. *Allergy Asthma Proc.* 2010; 31(2):158-160.
Rivard J, Lim HW. Ultraviolet phototherapy for pruritus. *Dermatol Ther.* 2005;18(4):344-354.

The images were produced while the author was a full time federal employee. They are in the public domain.

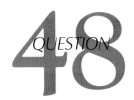
AFTER CHILDREN GET LACERATIONS OR STITCHES, HOW CAN I HELP PREVENT OR MINIMIZE SCARRING?

Christopher J. Miller, MD

One of the primary concerns of patients, parents, and health care providers confronted with traumatic lacerations is the final cosmetic appearance of the wound.[1] Excellent cosmetic outcomes depend largely on precise apposition of wound edges under minimal tension and avoidance of infection that can sabotage even the most precise surgical technique. Expedient care is a practical necessity in many pediatric patients, as younger children have difficulty cooperating during the procedure. After repair of the wound, primary interventions aim to improve the color and contour of the scar. An organized approach to lacerations can help to achieve consistently excellent results with efficient surgical technique.

Assessing the Wound and Determining the Plan of Care

The practitioner must first assess the wound to determine the anatomic structures affected by the injury, the relative risk for infection, the suitability of immediate repair of the wound, and the type of repair necessary. Injury to important anatomical structures, such as tendons, nerves, and arteries are often referred for specialist care and are beyond the scope of this chapter. This chapter will focus on superficial soft tissue injuries involving the epidermis, dermis, and/or subcutaneous fat.

The relative risk for infection increases if the source of injury is contaminated or if there is devitalized or necrotic tissue within the wound. Treatment with appropriate antibiotics and delayed closure is advised for wounds at high risk for contamination and infection, such as human or animal bites. Tetanus immunization status should be verified and updated as necessary. Crush injuries may result in a greater area of devitalized or necrotic tissue, which should be débrided prior to surgical repair.

Shearing injuries from sharp objects with no evidence of contamination have a low risk for either infection or necrotic tissue, and these clean lacerations are amenable to immediate repair. Based on the depth of the laceration, the degree of tension or motion at the site of the injury, and the complexity of the edges of the laceration, the practitioner will determine whether the wound requires a layered (ie, buried and cutaneous sutures) versus a simple closure (ie, cutaneous sutures only). In general, if the wound extends full thickness through the dermis, if the wound is in an area of high tension or repetitive motion, or if the edges of the laceration are scalloped or complex, a layered closure may produce a better long-term result.

Managing the Environment to Decrease Anxiety of the Child and Parents

Repairing lacerations of children requires more than surgical skills, since the practitioner must also manage the fears of the child and the anxiety of the parents. Key strategies include distraction techniques, maintaining a calm and controlled environment, and clear demonstration of efforts to minimize pain. Distraction with books, videos, music, jokes, or a variety of techniques may have a calming influence and help to divert the child's attention away from the injury. Decreasing traffic of personnel and minimizing surgical preparation in front of the child and parents will help to create as calm and controlled an environment as possible. Acquire all surgical supplies and prepare the surgical tray in an area remote from the child whenever possible. Before initiating the repair, have a clear conception of the surgical plan and meticulously organize the supplies and instruments necessary for every step of the procedure. Careful preoperative preparation pays dividends by reducing traffic in and out of the room and increasing efficiency during the procedure.

Achieving Anesthesia

Most children fear needles and have anxiety about pain during the procedure. The practitioner can use the time necessary to prepare the surgical supplies to initiate topical anesthesia and gain confidence from the child and parents that minimizing pain is a priority. Topical anesthesia with eutectic mixture of local anesthetics (EMLA) cream may eliminate the need for injectable anesthesia for superficial wounds or decrease the pain associated with injection of local anesthesia for wounds requiring layered closure. EMLA requires as long as 55 minutes for onset, limiting the practicality of its use.[2] Whether or not the anesthesia from EMLA is complete at the start of the procedure, patients and parents may derive psychological relief from its use.

Complete anesthesia is an absolute necessity, since the experience of pain will raise anxiety and decrease patient compliance. For most procedures, local injectable anesthesia will be necessary. Lidocaine 1% with epinephrine 1:100,000 is a common, commercially available preparation. Buffering the lidocaine with sodium bicarbonate at a ratio of 1:10 results in a more rapid and less painful onset of anesthesia.[3] Warming the anesthetic solution to body temperature, slow infiltration, and use of a narrow, 30-gauge needle will also minimize pain with injection. Ensure that anesthesia is complete in all areas of potential involvement during the procedure. While the onset of anesthesia is nearly immediate, it is often advantageous to allow several minutes for the child and parents to gain trust that the child will not experience any additional pain during the procedure.

Preparing the Wound for Closure

Once anesthesia is complete and the child recognizes that he or she will no longer experience pain, the wound can be prepared for closure. First, the wound is cleaned with an antiseptic and draped with sterile or clean drapes. More careful inspection of the wound will now be possible, since manipulation will not hurt the child. All visible foreign bodies should be removed and the wound should be irrigated with saline solution applied with pressure through a large syringe. Any devitalized or necrotic tissue should be sharply débrided.

Wound edges that are frayed, scalloped, or beveled will prevent precise approximation. Frayed and scalloped edges should be freshened with the scalpel to provide a straight, clean wound edge. Any bevel of dermis or fat at the wound edge should be freshened with the scalpel to produce a vertical face to the wound edge.

Simple Closure of Shallow and Uncomplicated Wounds

Superficial lacerations that do not extend full thickness through the dermis or small and uncomplicated full thickness lacerations in the areas with low tension may be repaired with a simple layer of cutaneous sutures. Common absorbable cutaneous sutures include fast-absorbing gut sutures, chromic gut, and vicryl rapide. Common nonabsorbable sutures include nylon and polypropylene. There is no difference in cosmetic outcome and complication rates between absorbable versus nonabsorbable sutures for repair of facial lacerations.[4]

Larger caliber sutures are more likely to leave scars with visible suture marks. More delicate sutures, such as 5-0 or 6-0, are ideal for wounds on the face. Wounds on the trunk and extremities will usually require a stronger suture, ranging from 3-0 to 5-0, depending on the relative degree of tension. Cutaneous sutures left in place for longer than 7 days commonly leave permanent scars, often called track marks (Figure 48-1). To optimize cosmesis, top sutures should be removed within 1 week. It is important to recognize that a wound has only 10% of its original tensile strength at 10 days after repair.[4] Therefore, a wound closed with a single layer of sutures remains very fragile at the ideal time for suture removal and is at increased risk for dehiscence.

Figure 48-1. Example of undesirable scar with track marks. The spread of the scar and unsightly track marks may have been avoided with more effective placement of buried dermal sutures.

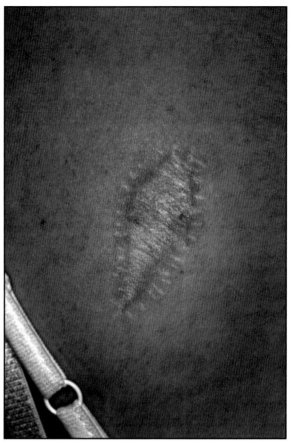

Alternative Methods of Approximating the Epidermal Wound Edges

Cyanoacrylates are tissue adhesives with some advantages over sutures in the repair of pediatric lacerations. Compared to sutures, they requires less time, are relatively painless, and do not require suture removal. Multiple studies have shown cosmetic results comparable to sutures wounds.[5] The majority of parents choose tissue adhesives and perceive them to cause less pain for their children.[6] Despite these perceived and real advantages, tissue adhesives should be limited to wounds with easily approximated edges or deeper wounds that have been approximated with buried dermal sutures. Practitioners should not rely on tissue adhesives if there is tension at the wound edges or if the wound will be subject to repetitive movement, such as over a joint.

Staples are particularly useful to repair wounds of the scalp, trunk, and extremities when saving time is essential. Compared to skin sutures, staples have been shown to provide a cosmetically acceptable scar for simple lacerations of the scalp and require less time for application.[7] Careful approximation of wound edges with deep sutures prior to stapling is advised, since staples do not allow as meticulous approximation as sutures. In addition, staples are more painful to remove than sutures, which may be problematic in pediatric patients.

Adhesive tapes such as steri-strips and butterfly bandages have a high rate of dehiscence and are not adequate for primary closure of wounds under tension.[6] They should be reserved as adjuncts to reinforce wounds before and after suture removal.

Layered Closure of Lacerations

To obtain optimal cosmetic results, deep, buried, dermal sutures will often be necessary. Common absorbable deep sutures include polyglactin (Vicryl), polyglycolic acid (Dexon), polydioxanone (PDS), and polyglyconate (Maxon). Indications for a layered wound closure include lacerations that have complicated edges, are located in areas of tension, and extend full thickness through the dermis. Buried subcutaneous sutures also eliminate dead space to prevent hematoma formation and accumulation of exudate. By approximating the dermis, deep sutures allow placement of superficial sutures with less tension, thereby decreasing the risk of infection and suture marks. Moreover, buried sutures maintain the majority of their tensile strength for 1 to 2 months, which helps to reduce spread of the scar as it matures during the immediate postoperative period.

Postoperative Care

Sutured and stapled wound should be covered with a thin layer of petrolatum ointment, a nonstick gauze, and a pressure dressing to help minimize bleeding for the first 24 hours postoperatively. Thereafter, the wound can be washed with soap and water, and a new, similar dressing can be applied daily for approximately 1 week. The dressing will help to protect the wound from gross contamination and speed the rate of re-epithelialization by maintaining occlusion. Wounds closed with tissue adhesives do not require a wound dressing and can be washed, but not soaked, daily.

To avoid suture marks, cutaneous sutures should be removed within 7 days. Sutures may be left for up to 2 weeks in areas under high tension, such as acral sites. Wounds closed in a simple fashion may be reinforced with adhesive tapes after suture removal, since there are no buried sutures to prevent dehiscence of the fragile scar.

Interventions to Improve the Scar After It Is Sutured

Sound surgical technique is the best approach to prevent an unsightly scar. Despite one's best efforts, scars in pediatric patients tend to spread, especially if the wound is sutured under tension. Postsurgical intervention may be helpful to improve scar appearance, especially color and contour of the scar. These same techniques can be used for nonsutured scars from trauma such as falling into a table. Patients may inquire about multiple over-the-counter scar treatment products, but minimal evidence supports their use. Patients should understand the wide disparity between the benefits advertised by manufacturers and the actual results from these products.[8] Of all over-the-counter scar treatments, silicone gel sheets are most likely to offer some benefit and can be used

Figure 48-2. Conservative intervention may improve scar appearance. (A) 16-year- old girl with hypertrophic scar 2 months after surgical repair. (B) Appearance 5 months later. Contour improved after injection with intralesional steroid. Scar has spread, which is common in pediatric patients.

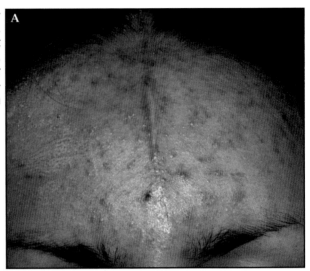

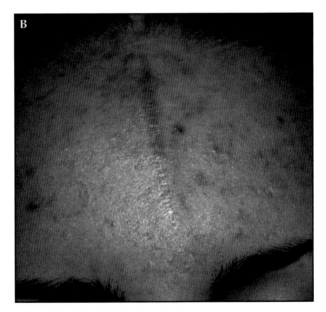

immediately after suture removal for 8 to 12 weeks. It is very challenging to get young children to keep silicone scar sheets on and the risk of choking hazard if they come off must be weighed in very young children.

Since the appearance of most scars will improve significantly after 2 to 3 months, it is often wise to delay intervention until assessment of the scar at that time. Conservative interventions may be helpful. If the scar is pink from telangiectasias, treatment with the pulse-dye laser may accelerate improvement in scar color. Scars with thick texture or hypertrophy may benefit from injections with intralesional steroids (Figure 48-2). The concentration and frequency of injection can be tailored according to the thickness of the scar. Thicker scars may require a higher concentration of intralesional steroid.

If these conservative measures do not improve the scar, scalpel-based scar revision may be necessary. Referral to a surgical specialist can be helpful.

With careful surgical technique and closer postoperative surveillance, children with lacerations can enjoy consistently excellent outcomes.

References

1. Singer AJ, Mach C, Thode HC Jr, Hemachandra S, Shofer FS, Hollander JE. Patient priorities with traumatic lacerations. *Am J Emerg Med.* 2000;18(6):683-686.
2. Hollander JE, Singer AJ. Laceration management. *Ann Emerg Med.* 1999;34(3):356-367.
3. Bartfield JM, Gennis P, Barbera J, Breuer B, Gallagher EJ. Buffered versus plain lidocaine as a local anesthetic for simple laceration repair. *Ann Emerg Med.* 1990;19(12):1387-1389.
4. Luck RP, Flood R, Eyal D, Saludades J, Hayes C, Gaughan J. Cosmetic outcomes of absorbable versus nonabsorbable sutures in pediatric facial lacerations. *Pediatr Emerg Care.* 2008;24(3):137-142.
5. Holger JS, Wandersee SC, Hale DB. Cosmetic outcomes of facial lacerations repaired with tissue-adhesive, absorbable, and nonabsorbable sutures. *Am J Emerg Med.* 2004;22(4):254-257.
6. Lloyd JD, Marque MJ 3rd, Kacprowicz RF. Closure techniques. *Emerg Med Clin North Am.* 2007;25(1):73-81.
7. Khan AN, Dayan PS, Miller S, Rosen M, Rubin DH. Cosmetic outcome of scalp wound closure with staples in the pediatric emergency department: a prospective, randomized trial. *Pediatr Emerg Care.* 2002;18(3):171-173.
8. Morganroth P, Wilmot AC, Miller C. Over-the-counter scar products for postsurgical patients: disparities between online advertised benefits and evidence regarding efficacy. *J Am Acad Dermatol.* 2009;61(6):e31-e47.

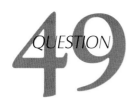
ARE THERE SKIN FINDINGS THAT ARE PART OF PARANEOPLASTIC SYNDROMES OR MARKERS OF RISK OF INTERNAL MALIGNANCY?

Randy Tang, MD and Warren R. Heymann, MD

A paraneoplastic syndrome is a disorder that is a consequence of a cancer but not directly caused by malignant cells; it is presumably triggered by an altered immune response to the associated tumor. Often the paraneoplastic syndrome alerts the clinician to the possibility of a remote neoplasm. This question summarizes several cutaneous paraneoplastic syndromes and other skin findings that are linked to internal malignancies in the pediatric population. The exact prevalence of cutaneous paraneoplastic syndromes in children is unknown owing to the rarity of occurrences, the complexity of the diseases, and the variation in presentation. Some skin findings are associated with a specific malignancy such as the relationship between juvenile xanthogranulomas (JXGs) with café-au-lait spots and juvenile myelomonocytic leukemia (JMML), while other cutaneous findings such as acanthosis nigricans (AN) can be a marker for a spectrum of conditions ranging from benign to malignant.

Dr. Helen O. Curth first proposed a set of criteria in 1976 to assess whether a cutaneous finding is a paraneoplastic phenomenon. Curth criteria requires that the skin rash be relatively uncommon, that it occurs concurrently or follows a parallel course with an underlying malignancy, that there exists a specific tumor site or cell type associated with the cutaneous disease, that there is a statistical association between the two processes, and that there may be a genetic association between the two disorders. Based on Curth criteria, several skin lesions or rashes in childhood should alert the clinician to a possible internal malignancy. A brief discussion of severe pruritus, AN, juvenile dermatomyositis (JDM), JXGs, paraneoplastic pemphigus (PNP), pyoderma gangrenosum (PG), and Sweet syndrome are detailed next.

Severe Pruritus

Severe intractable pruritus may be the initial presenting sign of hematological malignancies such as polycythemia vera, Hodgkin lymphoma, and non-Hodgkin lymphoma. The acute development of a generalized intense itch without the presence of a noticeable rash (especially in the absence of a history of atopy or xerosis) that does not improve with standard antipruritic therapies such as antihistamines should alert the clinician to the possibility of an internal malignancy. Typically, the itching spares flexural surfaces and is much more intense than that seen in atopic dermatitis. Occasionally, systemic symptoms such as fever, weight loss, and night sweats further support the presence of an internal (usually hematologic) malignancy. The severe pruritus often resolves with proper treatment of the malignancy.

Occasionally, severe pruritus may accompany a rash. For example, one reported case of severe pruritis was accompanied by prurigo nodules (which are firm, 1- to 3-cm nodules that may have a raised warty surface, overlying crusting or scaling, and characterized by intense itching), and this was the initial presenting sign in a teenager with lymphoma. Like other paraneoplastic skin rashes, the pruritus resolved when the underlying malignancy was treated appropriately. Finally, intractable pruritus may also be a manifestation of systemic mastocytosis, a disease that may transform into a hematological malignancy. Therefore, patients with severe pruritus of unclear etiology should be followed very closely.

Acanthosis Nigricans

AN, characterized by hyperpigmented, velvety thickening of the skin on intertriginous areas of the body, is most commonly associated with insulin resistance and obesity. The incidence of AN in the pediatric population has increased in conjunction with the increasing childhood obesity epidemic. Insulin and insulin-like growth factor-1 stimulate the growth of keratinocytes and dermal fibroblasts, resulting in the characteristic skin changes. In very rare cases, the appearance of AN in children heralds an underlying malignancy. In the absence of insulin resistance, the sudden appearance of AN involving atypical body sites such as palms, soles, or mucous membranes (particularly the lips and buccal mucosa) should raise concern for an underlying malignancy. Typically, malignant AN is also pruritic in nature. The few cases of pediatric paraneoplastic AN reported in the literature have been associated with Wilms tumor, osteogenic sarcoma, gastric carcinoma, and papillary thyroid carcinoma.[1] In these malignancies, the tumor cells produce growth factors that enhance keratinocyte and dermal fibroblast proliferation. In such cases, AN often resolves once the malignancy has been treated successfully.

Juvenile Dermatomyositis

JDM, clinically indistinguishable from adult-onset dermatomyositis (with the exception of a higher incidence of myositis ossificans), is an inflammatory disease of unclear etiology. JDM is characterized by proximal muscle weakness and cutaneous findings

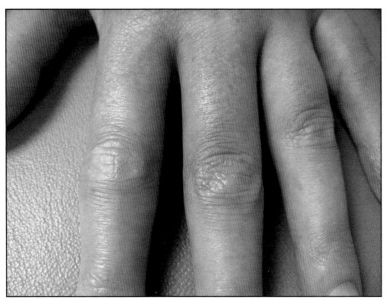

Figure 49-1. Red papules over the knuckles in a patient with dermatomyositis.

such as erythema of the eyelids with periorbital edema (heliotrope rash), erythematous to violaceous papules over the extensor aspects of the interphalangeal joints (Gottron papules; Figure 49-1) as well as elbows and knees (Gottron sign), and erythema of the neck and upper chest in a V-shaped distribution (shawl sign). While up to 33% of adults with dermatomyositis have an underlying malignancy, JDM as a paraneoplastic phenomenon has only been rarely reported in association with leukemia or lymphoma. In the absence of hepatosplenomegaly, lymphadenopathy, or a suggestive complete blood cell count, an extensive evaluation for malignancy in the pediatric population with JDM is not warranted, although continued clinical surveillance is prudent.

Juvenile Xanthogranulomas

JXGs are typically benign, asymptomatic red, yellow, or brown nodules composed of histiocytes of the non-Langerhans cell type that arise in infancy with a predilection for the head and neck. A child with neurofibromatosis-1 (NF-1), characterized by multiple café-au-lait macules and neurofibromas, who also has one or more JXGs is at a significantly higher risk of developing JMML (Figure 49-2).[2] While screening for JMML in NF-1 patients with multiple JXGs remains controversial because of the very low rate of such a paraneoplastic association, they should be followed very closely. The findings of hepatosplenomegaly, lymphadenopathy, or abnormalities on complete blood count should prompt the search for malignancy. Finally, there are case reports that detail the development of JMML in children with multiple JXGs without a history of NF-1 as well as rare reports of the sudden onset of multiple JXGs in patients with underlying acute lymphoblastic leukemia.

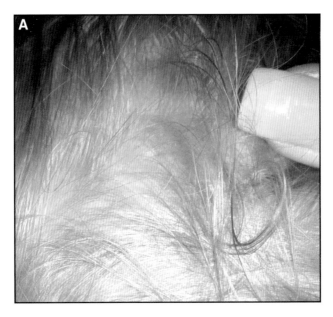

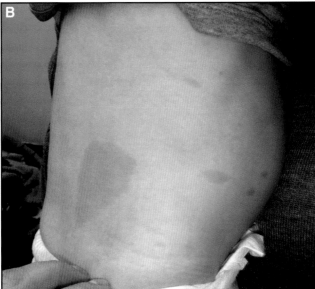

Figure 49-2. (A) JXG in the scalp. (B) Café-au-lait macules in the same patient with proven NF-I.

Paraneoplastic Pemphigus

PNP, an autoimmune mucocutaneous disease, is associated with non-Hodgkin lymphoma, thymoma, and Castleman disease in children. In many reported pediatric cases, PNP presented in the oral cavity as severe mucositis (involving the lateral tongue and vermilion most commonly) and as widespread cutaneous blisters, erosions, and ulcerations. The oral erosions are painful and often occur very early in the disease course. Erosions and subsequent crusting of the lips are typical and similar to that seen in patients with Stevens-Johnson syndrome, therefore, it is important to distinguish such patients from those with PNP by a complete history and physical examination as well as laboratory tests that include checking for herpes simplex virus and *Mycoplasma pneumoniae* titers.

In one study, 12 out of 14 pediatric patients with PNP had underlying Castleman disease,[3] which is a rare nonmalignant lymphoproliferative disorder that often manifests with systemic constitutional symptoms and enlarged lymphoid tissue at a single site or widespread throughout the body. Hypersecretion of the cytokine, interleukin-6, by lymph node germinal center B-cells accounts for the underlying etiology. Serum autoantibodies against plakin proteins are overproduced in the Castleman tumors and are responsible for the development of cutaneous lesions. While PNP may resolve with treatment of the underlying malignancy, patients with underlying Castleman disease have a very high mortality rate secondary to bronchiolitis obliterans.

Pyoderma Gangrenosum

PG appears as a large, deep ulceration, with a violaceous, scalloped, and undermined border. It is a neutrophilic dermatosis similar to Sweet syndrome (see below) and is classically associated with inflammatory bowel disease, rheumatoid arthritis, and other autoimmune diseases. PG, especially when presenting as an atypical bullous form, can occur as a paraneoplastic phenomenon in association with acute lymphoblastic leukemia and acute myelogenous leukemia. Several such cases have been described in the pediatric population.[4] Similar to Sweet syndrome, PG skin lesions often resolve with treatment of the leukemia.

Sweet Syndrome

Sweet syndrome (acute febrile neutrophilic dermatosis), characterized by the sudden onset of fever, leukocytosis with neutrophilia, and painful erythematous plaques over the trunks, limbs, and face, is thought to be a hypersensitivity reaction to viral, bacterial, or tumor antigens. In children, Sweet syndrome is classically associated with transient diseases such as respiratory tract infections and otitis media, as well as chronic diseases such as lupus erythematosus, vasculitis, immunodeficiency syndromes, aortitis, and chronic recurrent multifocal osteomyelitis. Additionally, Sweet syndrome can be a drug-related side effect (especially granulocyte colony stimulating factor and all-trans retinoic acid). In rare cases, Sweet syndrome presents as a paraneoplastic phenomenon. It has been reported in several pediatric patients with acute myelogenous leukemia. Cases have also been reported with acute lymphoblastic leukemia, juvenile chronic myelogenous leukemia, Fanconi anemia, and myelodysplastic syndrome.[5] In most pediatric paraneoplastic Sweet syndrome cases, the rash appeared only after the diagnosis of the malignant or premalignant disease was made and disappeared when the malignant disease entered remission.

Table 49-1

Paraneoplastic Skin Rashes and Associated Malignancies in the Pediatric Population

Acanthosis nigricans	Wilm's tumor, osteogenic sarcoma, gastric carcinoma, papillary thyroid carcinoma
Juvenile dermatomyositis	Leukemia, lymphoma
Juvenile xanthogranulomas with café-au-lait macules	Juvenile myelomonocytic leukemia
Paraneoplastic pemphigus	Castlemans disease, non-Hodgkins lymphoma, thymoma
Pyoderma gangrenosum	Acute lymphoblastic leukemia, acute myelogenous leukemia
Sweet syndrome	Acute myelogenous leukemia, juvenile chronic myelogenous leukemia, Fanconis anemia, myelodysplastic syndrome
Severe pruritus	Polycythemia vera, Hodgkins lymphoma, non-Hodgkin's lymphoma, systemic mastocytosis

Summary

Malignancies that manifest as skin rashes as part of paraneoplastic syndromes occur very rarely in children. The majority of these paraneoplastic skin rashes are associated with hematologic malignancies, notably leukemias and lymphomas. Knowledge of these associations is important for clinicians caring for children because the skin rash may be the initial presenting sign of an internal malignancy that otherwise might not be diagnosed until much later in the disease course. Table 49-1 summarizes the rare skin rashes in the pediatric population that are associated with malignancy.

References

1. Sinha S, Schwartz R. Juvenile acanthosis nigricans. *J Am Acad Dermatol.* 2007;57(3):502-508.
2. Zvulunov A, Barak Y, Metzker A. Juvenile xanthogranuloma, neurofibromatosis, and juvenile chronic myelogenous leukemia. World statistical analysis. *Arch Dermatol.* 1995;131(8):904-908.
3. Mimouni D, Anhalt GJ, Lazarova Z, et al. Paraneoplastic pemphigus in children and adolescents. *Br J Dermatol.* 2002;147(4):725-732.
4. Bakhshi S, Sethuramen G, Singh MK, Arya LS. Atypical pyoderma gangrenosum as a manifestation of childhood acute lymphoblastic leukemia. *Pediatr Dermatol.* 2005;22(6):543-545.
5. Hospach T, von den Driesch P, Dannecker GE. Acute febrile neutrophilic dermatosis (Sweet's syndrome) in childhood and adolescence: two new patients and review of the literature on associated diseases. *Eur J Pediatr.* 2009;168(1):1-9.

FINANCIAL DISCLOSURES

Dr. Faizan Alawi has no financial or proprietary interest in the materials presented herein.

Dr. Lisa Arkin has no financial or proprietary interest in the materials presented herein.

Dr. John C. Browning is a speaker for Galderma and a consultant for ViroXis.

Dr. Terri Brown-Whitehorn is involved in a research study with DBV pharmaceuticals looking at patch testing for oral desensitization.

Dr. Leslie Castelo-Soccio has no financial or proprietary interest in the materials presented herein.

Dr. Glen H. Crawford has no financial or proprietary interest in the materials presented herein.

Dr. Bhavik S. Desai has no financial or proprietary interest in the materials presented herein.

Dr. Magdalene Dohil has no financial or proprietary interest in the materials presented herein.

Dr. Lawrence F. Eichenfield is a consultant for Coria/Valeant, Galderma Labs, Johnson & Johnson, Ortho Dermatologics, Photocure, and Stiefel/GSK Company; is on the Advisory Board for Coria/Valeant; is an investigator for Galderma Labs, Johnson & Johnson, Ortho Dermatologics, Photocure, and Stiefel/GSK Company; and is a speaker for Coria/Valeant and Stiefel/GSK Company.

Dr. Dirk M. Elston has no financial or proprietary interest in the materials presented herein.

Dr. Brian T. Fisher receives research support from Pfizer Pharmaceuticals.

Dr. Ilona J. Frieden is a consultant for Pierre Fabre Dermatology.

Dr. Sheila F. Friedlander has no financial or proprietary interest in the materials presented herein.

Dr. Sarah M. Frioux has no financial or proprietary interest in the materials presented herein.

Dr. Maria C. Garzon has no financial or proprietary interest in the materials presented herein.

Dr. Warren R. Heymann has no financial or proprietary interest in the materials presented herein.

Dr. Paul J. Honig has not disclosed any relevant financial relationships.

Dr. Sharon E. Jacob has no financial or proprietary interest in the materials presented herein.

Dr. Christine T. Lauren has received grant from the Children's Medical Fund to use iPads as a distraction technique during pediatric procedures.

Dr. Moise L. Levy is a investigator for Pierre Fabre and Stiefel/GSK; was a speaker for Valeant; is a consultant for Valeant, Stiefel/GSK, and Galderma; is on the editorial board for *Archives of Dermatology;* and is editor for *Pediatric Dermatology, Up to Date.*

Dr. Erin F. Mathes has no financial or proprietary interest in the materials presented herein.

Dr. Patrick McMahon has no financial or proprietary interest in the materials presented herein.

Dr. Christopher J. Miller has no financial or proprietary interest in the materials presented herein.

Dr. Kimberly D. Morel has no financial or proprietary interest in the materials presented herein.

Dr. Adam Nabatian has no financial or proprietary interest in the materials presented herein.

Dr. Marissa J. Perman has no financial or proprietary interest in the materials presented herein.

Dr. Andres Pinto has no financial or proprietary interest in the materials presented herein.

Dr. Anna S. Salinas has no financial or proprietary interest in the materials presented herein.

Dr. Kara N. Shah has no financial or proprietary interest in the materials presented herein.

Dr. Randy Tang has no financial or proprietary interest in the materials presented herein.

Dr. James R. Treat has no financial or proprietary interest in the materials presented herein.

Dr. Joanne Wood has no financial or proprietary interest in the materials presented herein.

Dr. Albert C. Yan has no financial or proprietary interest in the materials presented herein.

Dr. Andrea L. Zaenglein has received a research grant from Astellas.

INDEX

ABCDE signs. *See* asymmetry, irregular borders, changing color, diameter, and enlargement signs
abscesses, 170, 171, 175, 239
acanthosis nigricans, 264
ACD. *See* allergic contact dermatitis (ACD)
acne
  hormonal therapy, 231
  infantile, 225–226
  management, 232
  mid-childhood, 226
  mild, initial therapy, 227
  mild-to-moderate, 231
  minocycline, 111
  moderate to severe, 232
  neonatal, 225
  oral antibiotics, 230
  preadolescent and adolescent, 227
  scars, blue skin pigmentation, 230
acquired melanocytic nevi, 51, 61
  in adolescent, 56
  benign, children, 57
  biopsy/excision, 58
  dysplastic nevus, 57
  eclipse, 55, 56
  with freckles, 55
  fried egg appearance, 57
  risk factors, 55
  on scalp, 55
acral nevi, 66
acyclovir, mucocutaneous dosing, 154
AD. *See* atopic dermatitis (AD)
adrenal tumors, 226
alanine aminotransferase (ALT), 90
allergic contact dermatitis (ACD), 132–133, 135
  children, diaper materials, 135
  diagnosis, 132
  irritant contact dermatitis, differentiating, 133
  nickel, 133, 134
  poison ivy, 132
  shoe materials, 136
  Toxicodendron genus plants, 133

allergic rhinitis/asthma, 159
allergic sensitization, 157–158
alopecia
  antidandruff shampoos, 219
  black dot tinea, 218
  kerion, 217
  non-scarring, 221
  psychological stress/nervousness, 219
  ringworm of scalp, 217
  scarring, 220
  selenium sulfide shampoo, 218
  telogen effluvium, 220
  traction, 220
  trichotillosis, 220
  types of, 217
ALT. *See* alanine aminotransferase (ALT)
amoxicillin
  arthritis, 202
  isolated facial nerve palsy, 202
  for Lyme disease, 199–201
  single/multiple erythema migrans lesion(s), 202
  for vulvar and perineal itching, 116
androgenetic alopecia, 217
anesthesia, 256, 257
angel's kiss, 24
angioedema, drug rashes, 92
angiotensin-converting enzyme inhibitors, 92
animals
  bites, 255
  flea treatments, 107
antibiotics
  for bacterial infection, 89
  B-lactams, macrolides for pustulosis, 92
  contact dermatitis, 134
  Lyme disease, clinical presentation, 202
  oral, 176
  purpuric lesions, 97
  SSLR, 91
  therapy, 117, 175
  topical, 134
  unnecessary exposures, 197